Visual Agnosia

Visual Agnosia

second edition

By Martha J. Farah

A Bradford Book
The MIT Press
Cambridge, Massachusetts
London, England

This book was set in Bembo by Graphic Composition, Inc.
Printed and bound in the United States of America.

Library of Congress Cataloging-in-Publication Data

Farah, Martha J.
Visual agnosia / by Martha Farah.—2nd ed.
  p.; cm.
"A Bradford book."
ISBN 0-262-06238-0 (hc: alk. paper) —ISBN 0-262-56203-0 (pbk : alk. paper)
1. Visual agnosia. 2. Visual perception. I. Title.
[DNLM: 1. Agnosia—physiopathology. 2. Form Perception—physiology. 3. Pattern Recognition, Visual. 4. Prosopagnosia. WL 340 F219v 2004]
RC394.V57F37   2004
616.8—dc22   2003059393

10 9 8 7 6 5 4 3 2 1

For Hermine Makman

Contents

Chapter 9

Chapter 10

Preface

When the first edition of this book came out in 1990, I joked that most authors spend a number of years working on a topic and then write a book about it, but I had written the book first and planned to then begin working on the topic. This was no exaggeration. It is a matter of record that my very first publication on object recognition or agnosia was the book! My backward, and some might say nervy, approach worked out surprisingly well. The agnosia case literature was an unmined resource, and experimental research on agnosia to answer questions about object recognition had barely begun. It seemed to me that the first order of business was simply reviewing and systematizing the case literature and posing some basic questions that could, in principle, be answered by such cases. A book was as good a way to do this as any. So I wrote *Visual Agnosia*.

Looking back at the first edition, it had an extremely high question-to-answer ratio. Many of the unanswered questions formed the basis for the next several years of my research: Are faces "special?" Is their geometry represented differently from that of other objects? Are there orthography-specific brain systems? How could they develop? Do "living things" constitute a special category for the visual system? For the semantic system?

In the fourteen years since the first edition came out, these and many other questions about visual object recognition have been addressed by myself and others around the world. Where before there were just a lot of interesting questions, now there is consensus on some answers, healthy differences of opinion on others, new questions, and plenty of solid science to make the second edition a very different book from the first.

My own contributions in the interim were undertaken with a very talented and congenial group of collaborators. In particular, four of my students played a major role in the research described here, and it is a pleasure to acknowledge their contributions. My former graduate student Shaun Vecera, now Associate Professor at the University of Iowa, took a set of general issues concerning attention, grouping, and early vision and translated them into a productive research program encompassing patient-based research, psychophysics, and computational modeling. The best thing I did for him as an advisor was move to Penn, leaving him to rely his own judgment and creativity. Thad Polk, a former postdoc and now Associate Professor at the University of Michigan, was the driving force behind our studies of perceptual processes in reading. In the course of building several computational models and conducting both behavioral and imaging experiments, Thad uncovered important new insights about the effects of experience on pattern recognition and also learned first-hand the meaning of "going postal." Former postdoc Jim Tanaka, now Professor of Psychology at the University of Victoria, took the lead in our work on parts and wholes in face recognition. Jim also saw the broader relevance of this work beyond face recognition and has made it one aspect of his multifaceted program of research on perceptual expertise. Paddy McMullen, another former postdoc now in Canada, where she is Associate Professor at Dalhousie University, was my partner in puzzlement for our initial studies of category-specific semantic impairments. She was able to get us past that stage with her thoughtful analysis and experimental rigor. Former postdocs Matt Kurbat, Cathy Reed, Sharon Thompson-Schill, and Lynette Tippett, graduate students Randy O'Reilly, Marcie Wallace, and Kevin Wilson, and research assistants Karen Klein, Karen Levinson, Carol Rabinowitz, and Matt Stallcup all worked with me on projects that were related in some way to the topic of this book, and their contributions are all gratefully acknowledged.

Much of the research reported here would have been impossible without the help of our agnosic subjects. These individuals worked with us in experiments that were often tedious and always difficult, designed as they were to elicit the subjects' agnosic impairments. I especially want to acknowledge the participation of Lincoln H., a remarkable person who has taught me much about visual agnosia, as well as experience, adaptability, and hope.

Barbara Murphy of MIT Press provided advice, encouragement, and an occasional kick in the pants, without which this book would probably still be a manuscript. Katherine Almeida expertly guided the book through production. I am grateful to them both. My colleague Russell Epstein at Penn and Tim Rogers of the MRC Cognition and Brain Unit in Cambridge, England read drafts of chapters and gave me their very knowledgeable and diplomatic advice, which I have tried to follow. Finally, my acknowledgments would not be complete without thanking three wise, generous and fun colleagues for their collaboration and tutelage in the area of visual object recognition, Todd Feinberg, Jay McClelland, and Mike Mozer.

Visual Agnosia

Chapter 1

Introduction

Virtually everything we know about the brain functions underlying human cognition has been learned by one of two methods: studying brain-lesioned patients and functional neuroimaging. The two methods tend to yield reassuringly consistent evidence. Yet they have significantly different strengths and weaknesses, to be discussed later in this chapter, and for this reason neither method is dispensable.

Disorders of visual object recognition following brain damage are known as visual agnosias. There is amazing diversity to the ways in which object recognition can break down, from visual form agnosia in which patients with normal acuity cannot recognize something as simple as a circle or a square, to topographic agnosia in which patients with normal face, object, and word recognition cannot recognize locales. In each case the patterns of preserved and impaired abilities put useful constraints on our theories of how the normal visual recognition system works.

1.1 A Brief History of Agnosia

For much of its history, the study of agnosia focused on the question of whether there *is* such a thing as agnosia. Researchers began with this most basic of questions, and perhaps in retrospect stayed with it too long, because the syndrome seemed so counterintuitive and contradictory. How could someone be able, in the words of Humphreys and Riddoch's (1987b) book title, *To See but Not to See?* Repeatedly over the years, the concept of visual agnosia has met with skepticism. First Bay (1953), and then Bender and Feldman (1972), argued that visual agnosia, in the sense of a selective impairment in visual recognition per se, does not exist. Bay proposed that the appearance of a selective impairment in object recognition was invariably the result of a combination of two more general characteristics of agnosic patients. First, he suggested that these patients always have subtle impairments in elementary visual functions, which may be less apparent under the conditions of standard tests of visual fields, acuity, and so on, than when they are being used for object recognition under natural conditions. Second, he claimed that these patients suffer from a general intellectual decline. According to Bay, impairments in elementary vision and general intelligence may occasionally conspire to produce disproportionate difficulties with object recognition, but there is no such thing as an impairment in object recognition per se. Bender and Feldman (1972) supported Bay's claims with a systematic review of a large number of neurological patients. They searched all of the patient records from a twenty-year period at New York's Mount Sinai Hospital and found relatively few cases with visual recognition difficulties. What they took to be more damaging to the concept of agnosia was the fact that all of these cases also had some significant elementary visual and/or general intellectual impairments.

Bay, and Bender and Feldman won over many influential neuropsychologists to their point of view on agnosia (e.g., Critchley, 1964; Teuber, 1968), but their skepticism was not shared by everyone. Even though a "pure" case of agnosia (a patient with impaired visual object recognition and perfectly normal elementary visual and intellectual capabilities) would disprove the skeptics' position, the absence of such a case does not prove it. Neuropsychologists know far too well that "nature's experiments" are executed rather sloppily, and they would have very little to study if they confined themselves to pure cases of anything. With this in mind, Ettlinger (1956) made the important point that finding a "pure" agnosic was not the only way to settle the issue empirically. Just as effective would be the demonstration that agnosic patients were no more impaired in their intellectual and elementary visual capabilities than many nonagnosic patients. He demonstrated that this was true by systematically assessing a variety of elementary visual functions in patients already screened for generalized intellectual decline. Although only one of his cases had a true agnosia, and this case did have elementary visual impairments, he found other patients with more severe elementary visual impairments who were not agnosic. More recently, De Haan, Heywood, Young, Edelstyn, and Newcombe (1995) carried out a more stringent test of Ettlinger's hypothesis with three severe visual agnosics and a more comprehensive and sophisticated battery of visual tests. Their data supported Ettlinger's conclusion that whatever elementary visual impairments the agnosic patients had, they were not the cause of the agnosia. Patients with equally impaired elementary visual function were not agnosic.

The impulse to "explain away" agnosia can be understood in terms of the theories of vision available to agnosia's skeptics in the mid-twentieth century. If one views object recognition as taking place in two relatively undifferentiated stages—(1) seeing the object and (2) associating general knowledge with the visual percept—then the only possible way to disrupt object recognition is by disrupting vision or general knowledge. If object recognition difficulties seem disproportionate to difficulties of vision or general knowledge (as is the case, by definition, with visual agnosia), then this must be due to a synergistic interaction of minor difficulties in both vision and general knowledge. However, with the advent of single unit recording in visual cortex (e.g., Gross, Rocha-Miranda, & Bender, 1972; Hubel & Weisel, 1962) and computational modeling of vision (e.g., Marr, 1982), a different view of visual object recognition emerged. According to this latter view, object recognition is accomplished by repeatedly transforming the retinal input into stimulus representations with increasingly greater abstraction from the retinal array and increasingly greater correspondence to invariant properties of objects in the physical world (see Farah, 2000). Within such a system, brain damage affecting just the later stages of vision would create a "pure" visual agnosia.

Eventually, neuropsychologists looked beyond the question of whether or not agnosia exists, to other questions about agnosia, including the possibility of different types of agnosia and their associated lesion sites. As the field of cognitive neuropsychology blossomed in the 1980s, researchers attempted to relate aspects of agnosia to theories of visual object recognition, and in the process to test those theories with data from agnosic patients (e.g., Farah, 1990; Humphreys & Riddoch, 1987b; Ratcliff & Newcombe, 1982). In the pages that follow, I will delineate a dozen or so distinct visual agnosic syndromes, and bring each of them to bear as evidence on the nature of visual object recognition. Examples of the questions to be addressed include: Are there different recognition modules, or subsystems, required for recognizing different kinds of stimuli (e.g., faces, common objects, printed words)? Does visual selective attention operate prior to object recognition, subsequent to it, or in parallel with it? Are the long-term visual memory representations underlying recognition implemented locally or in a distributed network?

1.2 Types of Agnosia

Taxonomizing may appear to be a rather atheoretical enterprise that would be better replaced by analysis of the phenomena of agnosia using cognitive theories. However, we must begin with issues of taxonomy because grouping the phenomena correctly, in any area of science, is a prerequisite for making useful theoretical generalizations about them. This is all the more important—and all the more difficult—in the study of agnosia because the entire database is comprised of single cases, no two of which are exactly alike. Therefore, much of the scientific work to be done in this field involves sorting these countless variable and unique cases into a tractable number of "natural kinds."

There is no standard taxonomy of agnosia. Everyone agrees that agnosic patients differ from each other in certain ways, but the question of which differences are differences of degree and which are differences of kind has not found a unanimous answer. On careful reading of patients' abilities and deficits, I find that many authors have grouped patients in unhelpful ways. Their implicit taxonomies misrepresent the basic empirical phenomena, both by overinclusive categories that blur theoretically important distinctions between different syndromes, and by overfractionation of syndromes, in which differences of degree are treated as differences of kind.

Most neuropsychologists follow Lissauer (1890) in distinguishing between the "apperceptive agnosias" and the "associative agnosias." According to Lissauer, apperceptive agnosias are those in which recognition fails because of an impairment in visual perception, which is nonetheless above the level of an elementary sensory deficit such as a visual field defect. Patients do not see objects normally, and hence cannot recognize them. In contrast, associative agnosias are those in which perception seems adequate to allow recognition, and yet recognition cannot take place. It is said to involve, in the oft-quoted phrase of Teuber (1968), a "normal percept stripped of its meaning."

In this respect, the apperceptive-associative distinction, as defined above, includes a significant assumption about the mechanisms of agnosia: that the underlying deficit in so-called associative agnosia lies outside of the modality-specific perceptual processing of the stimulus. Whether or not this is true is an important issue that will be discussed later. Nevertheless, the grouping of agnosics into two categories—those with prominent, easily noticed perceptual deficits and those without—does seem to be empirically valid.

Within these two broad categories there is tremendous variation. For example, among the patients who have been labeled "apperceptive" are those who cannot discriminate a circle from a square, those who can recognize any one object but cannot see other objects presented at the same time, and those whose difficulty with object recognition is manifest only with objects presented at unusual orientations. Among the patients who have been labeled "associative" are those whose impairment is confined to specific categories of visual stimulus such as faces, places, or printed words, as well as those with across-the-board recognition impairments and those who seem impaired only when naming a visually presented object. The organization of this book reflects my attempt to find a happy medium between lumping distinct syndromes together and splitting the phenomena into an unmanageable and unnecessary number of separate categories. Each of the next eight chapters describes a type of agnosia, along with its relations to theories of normal visual function.

1.3   Patient-Based Cognitive Neuroscience in the Age of Imaging

The first edition of this book was written one methodological revolution ago, just before functional neuroimaging transformed cognitive neuroscience. At that time, everything we knew about the neural bases of high-level vision in humans came from studies of patients. It was therefore particularly exciting to work through the rich database of clinical studies in search of insights about normal object recognition, knowing that such insights lay waiting there and, at the time, only there.

The situation is very different now. Neural systems can be visualized as they perform their functions under experimentally controlled conditions in normal subjects. This capability revolutionized all areas of cognitive neuroscience, and greatly expanded our understanding of high-level vision in the course of just a decade of research. It therefore bears asking: Why study visual agnosia now that functional neuroimaging is available? The answer to this question involves an accounting of the strengths and weaknesses of imaging and patient-based cognitive neuroscience.

An obvious weakness of patient-based research is that naturally occurring lesions do not respect anatomical or functional boundaries. Such messiness would be less of a problem if all possible sizes and shapes of these messy lesions occurred, because different patients with overlapping lesions might permit inferences about the functions of common and distinct subregions, but this is not the case; strokes, head injury, and other etiologies of brain damage have characteristic lesions, and many possible lesion configurations do not occur. The greatest advantage of functional neuroimaging is its ability to compensate for this weakness. Although some areas of the brain are better visualized with current imaging techniques than others, imaging is hands-down the better way to probe the functions of specific anatomical regions.

Functional neuroimaging has the additional advantage of studying normal brains, which are the subject of interest. With patient-based research we are operating one inferential step away from this subject. Of course, the behavior of a damaged system is related in systematic ways to the function of the intact system. But "systematic" does not mean "simple": reorganization following injury can greatly complicate our inferences about normal function (Farah, 1994). An additional problem with rare disorders, including most of the agnosias, is that patients provide no more than an existence proof that a certain dissociation is possible, and hence that the inferred neurocognitive organization exists. In the early days of cognitive neuroscience this was a minor worry, because of the implicit assumption that all normal human brains were wired in basically the same way. However, as our field finally begins to grapple with individual differences (Thompson, Cannon, Narr, van Erp, Poutanen, Huttunen, Lonnqvist, Standertskjold-Nordenstam, Kaprio, Khaledy, Dail, Zoumalan, & Toga, 2001; Hamer, 2002), we want to know whether the functional organization inferred from one patient applies to all humans or is just one variant. Does everyone use separate systems to recognize faces and non-face objects, or just a subpopulation, who will become prosopagnosic after certain patterns of brain damage? The ability to analyze individual subjects' images allows us to address this question by finding out what proportion of subjects recruits measurably different brain regions for face and object recognition.

In weighing the advantages and disadvantages of patient-based and imaging research, there is one other drawback to patient-based research that is often overlooked: the difficulty of interlaboratory verification. Findings from patients with rare disorders like agnosia cannot be pursued by any scientist with an alternative hypothesis or a good idea for a follow-up study. This is unavoidable, at least to a degree. When a patient agrees to work with one researcher, he is not making himself available to any scientist in the field willing to travel to him at any point in the future. However, the problem is often compounded by researchers who develop a possessiveness about "their" patients. This practice is at least as dehumanizing to the patient as offering to put them in contact with other researchers, and it has impeded progress in our field. Imaging studies are much more replicable, in that a finding from one imaging lab can in principle be pursued by any other imaging lab.

These advantages of imaging over patient-based research make an impressive list. If we were to play a variant of the childhood game "would you rather" (be rich or beautiful, fly like a bird or read minds . . .) with imaging and patient-based methods, I'd be inclined to take the imaging. Happily, we do not have to choose. Patient-based methods have their own strengths, which complement those of imaging. As a result, the combination of the two approaches is more powerful than the sum of its parts.

The great advantage of studying patients is the ability to test hypotheses about mechanism. The goal of most cognitive neuroscience research to understand *how* intelligent behavior is accomplished. We are trying to describe the causal chain of events that intervene between stimulus and response. We share this goal with a number of other disciplines, from molecular neuroscience to cognitive psychology. What distinguishes these disciplines is the level of description within which they cast their hypotheses about mechanism.

The mechanistic hypotheses of cognitive neuroscience concern the information-processing functions of macroscopic neural systems. This level of description includes, at the more microscopic end of the range, the emergent behavior of populations of neurons. It is this population behavior, during learning, normal function, and after damage, that does the explanatory "work" in the computational models described in this book (e.g., models of the word superiority effect, covert face recognition, optic aphasia, and selective semantic memory impairments). At the more macroscopic end of the cognitive neuroscience level of description are models that delineate distinct information processing components and their interrelations, such as the division of labor between form perception from static spatial cues and form from motion, and between face and object recognition.

Our methods deliver information that is useful for testing hypotheses at this level of description. Current imaging techniques reveal distinguishable activations at about this scale, and the relatively more fine-grained dissociations among abilities after brain damage can also be described at this level. However, images and lesions are very different in their ability to answer questions about mechanism. Only the lesion method can reveal the causal relations among brain systems.

Imaging data are fundamentally correlational; they tell us that this area becomes active when that cognitive process is being performed. They do not tell us what causal role, if any, is played by an activation observed in this way. Not every activation is part of a causal pathway; representations may become active, in a given task context, either because they are causally involved in performing the task or because they have become associated with other representations that are causally involved. Although it may seem odd to think of the brain as activating unnecessary systems, I suspect that superfluous or only marginally useful activity is very common, and perhaps the norm. Try the following low-tech demonstration of this point: Glance at the bottom of this page and count the letters in the last word. Notice that you read and understood the word even though it was not part of your assignment. Indeed, the same thing will happen even if you *try* not to read the word. Phonological and semantic representations are so highly associated with orthographic representations that they are activated even when not necessary. This example of associated activity is intentionally obvious, but the issue is not trivial when the activated systems are less open to introspection and less well characterized cognitively.

To tease apart causal and merely associated systems, and characterize the information-processing function of each of those systems, we need to reach in and tinker. Only by seeing the consequences of removing or disabling different candidate systems can we infer their role in producing a given behavior. Of course, with human brains we do not "tinker." Instead, we examine the effects of naturally occurring brain damage.

How can patient-based research determine which activated systems play a causal role in implementing an ability, and which are merely associated? To answer this question, let us return to the example of unnecessary but associated activity when counting the letters in a word. Imagine that this task has been carried out in a scanner, and consistent with introspection, areas subserving visual-spatial attention are activated (as they are in counting tasks), and areas subserving orthography, phonology, and semantics are activated (as they are when words are processed). We now want to answer the question: which of these activations play a causal role in implementing letter counting, and which are merely associated? We can find out by testing patients with lesions in each of these systems on the letter counting task.

Patients with disorders of visual-spatial attention, including the dorsal simultanagnosics of chapter 3, will have difficulty with the letter counting task. This is consistent with the hypothesis that counting visual stimuli requires marking them attentionally; the movement of visual-spatial attention from item to item is not merely an associated but unnecessary process. In contrast, patients with orthographic impairments (e.g., the pure alexic patients of chapter 4), phonological impairments, or semantic impairments (e.g., the optic aphasics and semantic agnosics of chapters 8 and 9) will be able to perform the task. This is consistent with the hypothesis that the lexical processes that were reliably activated in the scanner are not in fact necessary for the behavior.

The information that patients provide goes beyond simply classifying systems as necessary or not necessary. It can also distinguish different types of processing and delineate multiple parallel chains of processing that enable a behavior. Patterns of activation in functionally parallel systems do not tell us which activations are part of the same or different pathways, or what the unique information-processing nature of each system is. By contrast, through interrupting processing at various loci we can infer just these properties of the system, through a procedure akin to trouble-shooting.

The cognitive neuroscience of object recognition has already benefited from the interplay of patient-based and imaging methods. Initial attempts to investigate visual recognition using functional neuroimaging suffered from a lack of specific hypotheses and were correspondingly quite variable in matching experimental and baseline conditions. Many studies consisted of simply scanning subjects while they viewed pictures or performed tasks with assorted stimuli and fixation points. No wonder that, in the aggregate, this sizable literature succeeded only in establishing that visual object recognition involves the posterior half of the brain (Farah & Aguirre, 1999)! However, this changed as imagers began to test specific hypotheses about visual recognition, most of which came from the patient literature. For example, prosopagnosia and topographic agnosia suggested specific hypotheses concerning specialization in ventral visual areas, and along with more specific hypotheses came more theoretically constrained experimental designs. Imaging in turn clarified the degree of segregation among specialized recognition systems, which of course are never neatly dissociated by naturally occurring lesions.

It has recently become possible to combine imaging and patient-based research in a powerful new way, by imaging patients while they engage in the processes of interest. This approach poses many additional technical challenges beyond those of imaging a normal brain (Price & Friston, 2003), but is also uniquely well suited to understanding the anatomical and mechanistic bases of cognition. Although as yet undeveloped, the functional imaging of visual agnosics will undoubtedly play an increasingly dominant role in the cognitive neuroscience of high-level vision.

Chapter 2

Visual Form Agnosia

The term "apperceptive agnosia" has been used to mean any failure of object recognition in which perceptual impairments seem clearly at fault, despite relatively preserved sensory functions such as acuity, brightness discrimination, and color vision. It has been applied to an extremely heterogeneous set of patients who seem unlikely to share a single underlying impairment. In the first edition of this book, I reserved the term "apperceptive agnosia" for one particular syndrome, to which this label has most frequently been applied, and added a parenthetical "narrow sense" to signal the difference between this usage and the more general one. Clarity is probably better served, however, by a more distinct label, and so I propose to adopt the alternative term "visual form agnosia," introduced by Benson and Greenberg (1969).

2.1   Visual Form Agnosia: A Case Description

Benson and Greenberg (1969) touch on many of the essential features of this syndrome in the following description of Mr. S, a young man who suffered accidental carbon monoxide poisoning.

Visual acuity could not be measured with a Snellen eye chart, as he could neither identify letters of the alphabet nor describe their configuration. He was able to indicate the orientation of a letter "E," however, and could detect movement of a small object at standard distance. He could identify some familiar numbers if they were slowly drawn in small size on a screen. He could readily maintain optic fixation during fundoscopic examination, and optokinetic nystagmus was elicited bilaterally with fine, 1/8 inch marks on a tape. . . . Visual fields were normal to

10 mm and 3 mm white objects, and showed only minimal inferior constriction bilaterally to 3 mm red and green objects. . . .

The patient was able to distinguish small differences in the luminance (0.1 log unit) and wavelength (7–10 mu) of a test aperture subtending a visual angle of approximately 2 degrees. While he could detect these differences in luminance, wavelength, and area, and could respond to small movements of objects before him, he was unable to distinguish between two objects of the same luminance, wavelength, and area when the only difference between them was shape.

Recent and remote memory, spontaneous speech, comprehension of spoken language, and repetition were intact. He could name colors, but was unable to name objects, pictures of objects, body parts, letters, numbers, or geometrical figures on visual confrontation. Yet he could readily identify and name objects from tactile, olfactory, or auditory cues. Confabulatory responses in visual identification utilized color and size cues (a safety pin was "silver and shiny like a watch or a nail clipper" and a rubber eraser was "a small ball"). He identified a photograph of a white typewritten letter on a blue background as "a beach scene," pointing to the blue background as "the ocean," the stationery as "the beach," and the small typewriter print as "people seen on the beach from an airplane."

He consistently failed to identify or to match block letters; occasionally he "read" straight line numbers, but never those with curved parts. He could clumsily write only a few letters (X, L) and numbers (1, 4, 7), but often inverted or reversed these. Although he could consistently identify Os or Xs as they were slowly drawn, or if the paper containing them was moved slowly before him, he was unable to identify the very same letters afterwards on the motionless page. He was totally unable to copy letters or simple figures, and he could neither describe nor trace the outline of common objects. . . .

He was unable to select his doctor or family members from a group until they spoke and was unable to identify family members from photographs. At one time he identified his own face in a mirror as his doctor's face. He did identify his own photograph, but only by the color of his military uniform. After closely inspecting a scantily attired magazine "cover girl," he surmised that she was a woman because "there is no hair on her arms." That this surmise was based on flesh color identification was evident when he failed to identify any body parts. For example, when asked to locate her eyes he pointed to her breasts. . . . (pp. 83–85)

In summary, the patient had seemingly adequate elementary visual functions and general cognitive ability, and yet he was dramatically impaired on the simplest forms of shape discrimination. Indeed, this patient was described as appearing blind to casual observers (Efron, 1968). Let us relate the findings in this case to the others in the literature.

2.2   *Visual Form Agnosia: Some Generalities*

Visual form agnosia is a relatively rare syndrome, although the similarity
of a number of other reported patients to Mr. S suggest that it is a useful
category. Other visual form agnosics include the cases of HC (Adler, 1944;
Sparr, Jay, Drislane, & Venna, 1991), ES (Alexander & Albert, 1983), Mr. S
(Efron, 1968; Benson & Greenberg, 1969), RC (Campion & Latto, 1985;
Campion, 1987), Schn. (Gelb & Goldstein, 1918; translated by Ellis,
1938), and X (Landis, Graves, Benson, & Hebben, 1982), and DF (Milner, Perrett, Johnston, et al., 1991).

As was true for Mr. S, visual field defects do not seem responsible for
the visual problems of the other patients in this category. Visual fields are
either normal or sufficiently preserved that visual field defects do not seem
an adequate explanation of their visual difficulties. In all cases acuity is either normal or sufficient for recognition, and in most cases color vision is
roughly normal. Maintaining fixation of a visual target was possible for
all but one of these cases (Alexander & Albert, 1983), and was reported
difficult for one other (Adler, 1944). In the three cases in which depth perception was explicitly reported, it was either intact or recovered while the
patient was still agnosic. Motion perception was intact in some cases, although most did not report any specific tests of movement perception.

In striking contrast to their roughly intact visual sensory functions,
visual form agnosics are severely impaired at recognizing, matching, copying, or discriminating simple visual stimuli. These impairments are not
subtle: Typical examples of patients' errors on such tasks include calling the
numeral 9 "a capital A" (Adler, 1944), a circle "a lot of dots" (Campion,
1987), or being unable to discriminate simple shapes such as "Xs" from
"Os" (Benson & Greenberg, 1969; Milner et al., 1991). Figure 2.1 shows
the attempts of two of these patients to copy simple forms. Figure 2.2
shows the stimuli used in two shape-matching tasks that Mr. S was unable to perform. In the first task, pairs of rectangles with the same total area
were shown to the patient, and his task was to judge whether they had the
same shape or different shapes. In the second task, he was asked to match
a sample stimulus to one of four other stimuli that had the same shape.

The case reports give a few additional clues to the nature of these patients' perception of the visual world. For some patients it was mentioned
that figures made of dots were harder to recognize than figures made of

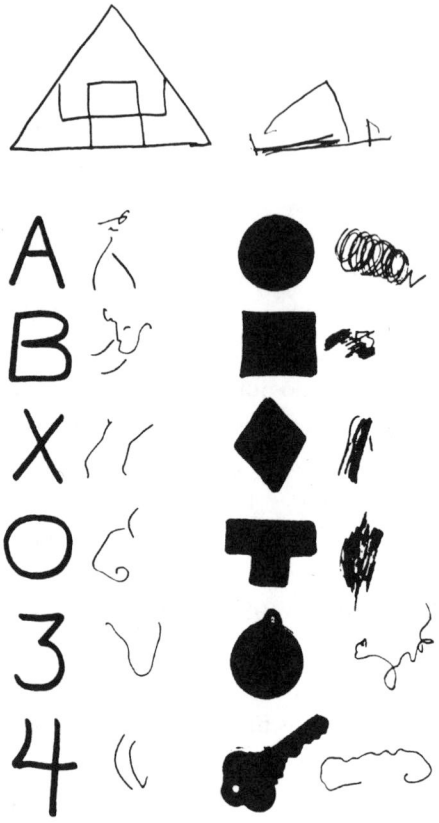

Figure 2.1
Copies of a geometric form by H. C. (*top*) and simple shapes, numbers, and letters by Mr. S (*bottom*).

solid lines, and curved lines were more difficult to perceive than straight. In two of the reports it was mentioned that the patients did not seem to perceive objects as solid forms or even surfaces in three dimensions: Adler (1944, p. 252) says of her patient, "At first she perceived contours only. For example, during the second week she called a nickel and a round silver compact each 'a key ring.'" Gelb and Goldstein (Ellis, 1938, p. 318) state that "All drawings in perspective were utterly meaningless for this patient. A circle tilted away from him was invariably described as an ellipse."

Recognition of real objects is also impaired but is somewhat better than recognition of "simple" stimuli. This appears to be due to the wider set of available cues to the identity of real objects, particularly color. The

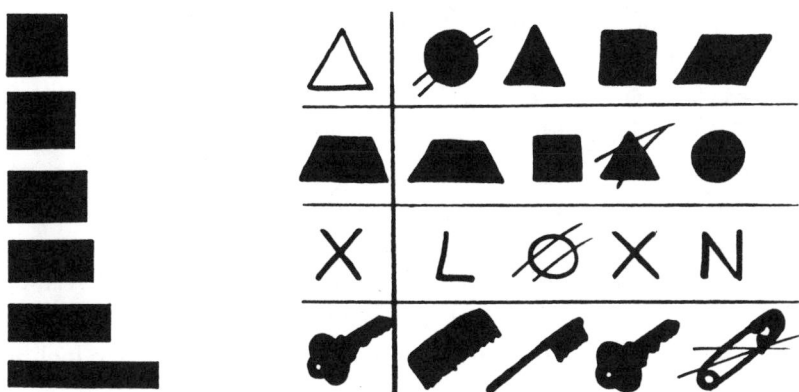

Figure 2.2
The shape-matching ability of an apperceptive agnosic patient. On the left is a set of rectangles matched for overall area, which were presented pairwise to Mr. S to be judged same or different in shape. He was unable to discriminate all but the most distinctive, and made errors even with these. On the right are a set of rows containing a target shape (*right*) and a set of four choices to be matched with the target shape. Mr. S's answers are marked.

patients' identifications of objects are typically *inferences,* made by piecing together color, size, texture, and reflectance clues. Mr. S's reliance on these properties is apparent from Benson and Greenberg's recounting of his attempts to recognize the safety pin and the picture of the typed letter. They also report that he "could select similar objects from a group only if there were strong color and size clues; after training he could name several familiar objects but failed to do so if their color and size qualities were altered. Thus he failed to identify a green toothbrush that was substituted for a previously named red toothbrush. He also called a red pencil "my toothbrush" (p. 84). RC was reported to use "features of objects, such as their color or whether they were shiny or not. He could also recognize the 'texture' of objects. If encouraged, he could often make an accurate guess about the nature of objects from such cues" (Campion, 1987, p. 209). Landis et al. (1982) report similar strategies in their patient, X: "He once mentioned being on the 14th floor of the hospital. Asked how he knew, he replied "It's the only one having red exit doors." Adler's patient, too, was said to recognize objects by "a process of adding up visual impressions," and often used color to guess the identity of objects, mistaking vanilla ice cream for scrambled eggs and a piece of white soap for a piece of paper (p. 252).

Motion of the object to be recognized appears to be helpful to some of these patients. Not surprisingly, it was helpful only to those subjects who had large visual fields, since a moving object would quickly pass out of view for patients with very narrow visual fields. ES recognized objects best when they were "alone and moving (e.g. identifying birds or planes flying at a great distance . . .)" (Alexander & Albert, 1983, p. 408). Motion helped Mr. S to segregate objects from their surround: "Mr. S can point with his finger to an object which is held before him. He can do this efficiently only if the object is moved before his eyes. If it is stationary he does not appear to know what object he has been asked to look at; his eyes randomly scan the entire room and he appears to be 'searching'" (Efron, 1968, p. 156). Motion also aided Mr. S's perception of form. Efron reports that "When I outlined a circular figure repeatedly with a pencil he was apparently able to see the shape. For a brief instant his face lit up with pleasure and he claimed that he saw the circle. A few minutes later, under static conditions, he was unable to identify the same object" (p. 159). Benson and Greenberg (1969) found that this patient was better able to recognize shapes that were moved slowly in front of him, and also that he could recognize shapes while they were being drawn, either with ink on paper (p. 83) or with a point of light on a screen (p. 85). Adler did not formally test the role of motion in HC's recognition abilities, but remarked that, at the movies, "the accompanying voices and her observation of movements contribute to her understanding" (p. 253). Landis et al. (1982) tested X's recognition of written material moved in front of the patient and reported that movement did not help. However, this patient normally recognized letters and words with the help of a tracing strategy, which would be foiled by stimulus movement. Therefore, the appropriate comparison would have been between moving and stationary stimuli when tracing strategies were prevented. However, like Mr. S, this patient "recognized words traced letter by letter in the air in front of him and did this much faster than any observers" (p. 522).

2.3   Inferring the Functional Locus of Impairment

Two account have been offered of the underlying nature of the impairment in visual form agnosia. The first was inspired by the observation that at least some visual form agnosics have "peppery" scotomas throughout their visual fields. Campion and Latto (1985) suggested that the general degradation of vision resulting from such visual field deficits could have a disproportionate effect on global form perception. This account has the appeal of parsimony, in postulating a simple, low-level impairment whose emergent effects include a loss of form perception. However, it is not clear by what mechanism such an effect would emerge. Why would the perception of simple, geometric forms, such as the rectangles shown in figure 2.2, be so profoundly disrupted by a peppery mask? Why would such a mask make it so hard to trace past a break in a line? And wouldn't the effect of a given mask vary according to stimulus size, an effect that has not been noted in the literature? If anything, the deletion of many random bits of a geometric figure would seem to encourage greater reliance on global shape properties such as "good continuity," rather than inducing a slavish reliance on local bits of contour.

Vecera and Gilds (1998) carried out an experiment with normal subjects that was designed to test this interpretation of visual form agnosia. Using the influence of global shape on attentional allocation as a measure of form perception, they compared the effect of two different stimulus manipulations: superimposing a peppery mask on the stimulus display, and removing the most salient grouping cues from the stimulus display. They found that the former had no effect on the pattern of subjects' reaction times, whereas the latter eliminated the shape effect. They concluded that peppery scotomas are not sufficient to explain the impairments of visual form agnosics. This conclusion was later challenged by Abrams and Law's (2002) finding that more severe degradation of the visual displays by peppery masks did eliminate the effects of shape on attentional allocation. However, they also report that their subjects were nevertheless able to perceive the shapes accurately, suggesting that the peppery mask hypothesis may be more relevant to explaining the attentional effects per se than the more general failure of shape perception in visual form agnosia.

The alternative hypothesis, implicit in the comparison condition of Vecera and Gilds's (1998) simulating peppery scotomas, is that a grouping process, distinct from the perception of local features, has been damaged. From the Gestalt psychologists of the early twentieth century to contemporary computational theories of vision (e.g., Sajda & Finkel, 1995), the grouping of local features on the basis of such perceptual properties as

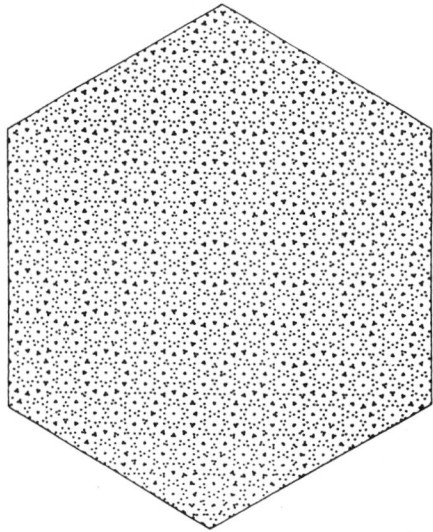

Figure 2.3
A demonstration of grouping processes at work. The shifting, scintillating patterns seen
here are the result of rivalrous grouping processes.

proximity, similarity, and good continuity has been treated as a fundamental stage in visual shape perception. The shifting, scintillating structure apparent in figure 2.3 is the result of grouping processes actively
organizing the local elements of the figure into alternative global struc-
tures. The "grouping hypothesis" of visual form agnosia (Farah, 1990)
takes this dissociation at face value, and infers that grouping is a functionally and anatomically separate visual function, distinct from perception of
local visual properties.

2.4   From Stuff to Things: The Emergence of Object Shape

Early vision has been characterized as representing "stuff" rather than
"things" (Adelson & Bergen, 1991), meaning that the visual system initially extracts information about local visual properties before computing
the larger scale structure of the image. In many ways, visual form agnosia
can be described as preserved stuff vision in the absence of thing vision.
What is striking about visual form agnosia is the complex nature of the
stuff that can be represented in the absence of things. The perception of

depth, velocity, acuity, and especially color (as opposed to wavelength), which are at least roughly intact in many visual form agnosics, requires considerable cortical computation (see Farah, 2000, chap. 2 for a review). These computations yield a kind of rich but formless visual goo, which requires some additional and separately lesionable grouping process to represent objects.

The process by which "things" emerge has been the subject of intense study within the vision sciences. In the 1980s and continuing in the 1990s, a central issue in computational vision research was the nature of the shape primitives that are first computed from the image. To continue with the terminology of the grouping hypothesis, the local shape information could initially be grouped into larger scale elements of contour, surface, or three-dimensional volumetric shape. In the early and influential model of vision proposed by Marr (1982), local features are first grouped into contours (the "full primal sketch"), from there into surfaces (the "two-and-a-half-D sketch"), and finally into volumetric primitives (the "three-D model"). More recently, a Bayesian approach to grouping (or image segmentation, as it is typically called in the literature) has proven capable of extracting things from stuff by using a set of probabilistically reliable cues to objecthood (Knill & Richards, 1996). This approach operates according to a kind of "any which way you can" principle, combining all potentially diagnostic features of the image to arrive at correct groupings, and is not concerned with whether the feature is primarily diagnostic of continuous contour, surface, or volume.

Visual form agnosics lack the ability to group local visual elements into contours, surfaces, and objects. Selectively preserved contour perception with impaired surface and volume perception, or preserved contour and surface perception and selectively impaired volume perception have never been reported. This is not strictly inconsistent with approaches which hypothesize a hierarchy of these different shape primitives. Perhaps a dissociation among these abilities is simply neurologically, unlikely given the etiologies of naturally occurring brain damage, or perhaps such a dissociation will be observed in the future. In the meantime, however, existing impairments in grouping seem most consistent with the simultaneous extraction of contour, surface, and volumetric shape information, which is characteristic of the Bayesian approach to image segmentation.

2.5   Form-from-Motion

The dramatic dissociation between the recognition of static and moving forms hints at another distinction between components of the normal visual system. Recall how Mr. S's face "lit up with pleasure" when he saw a circle being drawn and was able to recognize it; whereas a few minutes later, without the motion of the pencil, he was unable to identify the same circle. This and the many other descriptions of improved perception of moving shapes, and improved or even normal perception of motion path shape in visual form agnosics, suggests a residual spared pathway to shape perception. Specifically, it suggests that the derivation of form based on *spatiotemporal* factors, such as the correlations among the motions of a rigid body's local elements or the shape of a path traced in time, is independent of the derivation of form based on purely *spatial* factors such as proximity. This accords well with the results of more recent investigations of shape and motion processing in the primate brain, using single cell recording, and of functional neuroimaging in humans.

Both sources of evidence support the existence of anatomically separate pathways mediating the perception of static and moving forms. A ventral pathway, from occipital to inferotemporal cortex, is involved in static shape perception, whereas a different and more dorsal pathway mediates the perception of motion and of form-from-motion (Plant, Laxer, Barbaro, Schiffman, & Nakayama, 1993). The existence of two pathways does not necessarily imply two sets of shape representations, since the two pathways process different cues to shape or group local features by purely spatial versus spatiotemporal relations. Indeed, there is evidence that the two pathways share the same end point: Sary, Vogel, and Orban (1993) found that the shape preferences of neurons in inferotemporal cortex were invariant over three different cues to shape, including both luminosity cues and motion cues.

2.6   Visuomotor Function in Visual Form Agnosia

Movement plays another role in the perceptual abilities of some visual form agnosics, in their use of visually guided self-movement. The ability to "follow" a contour with a hand movement seems to have been preserved in number of cases. This was the most famous and controversial aspect of

Gelb and Goldstein's (1918) case, who traced the contours of stimuli using both head and hand movements. With sufficient time he was able to read most print by executing "a series of minute head and hand movements. He 'wrote' with his hand what his eyes saw. He did not move the entire hand, as if across a page, but 'wrote' the letters one over another, meanwhile 'tracing' them with head movements" (Ellis, 1938, p. 317). Gelb and Goldstein made several important observations about Schn.'s tracing behavior that shed light on the nature of his visual abilities as well as the functional role played by tracing: "If prevented from moving his head or body, the patient could read nothing whatever. . . . His movements led to reading only if they corresponded to normal writing movements. If required to trace a letter the 'wrong' way, he was quite at a loss to say what letter it was. . . . If a few cross-hatching marks were drawn across the word, he followed these when he reached them and consequently lost all sense of what the word was . . . the scratches 'derailed' him and he was unable to rediscover the correct path. . . . If the scratches were made with a different colored pencil, no difficulty was encountered; the same held for very thick letters and very thin scratches. . . . It may be said that his tracing was quite 'planless', if by plan we mean guidance based on an antecedent grasp of the structure of the object to be traced. If the drawing given him to be traced were, like a circle, of such a character that he had one route to follow, the result was always successful. Not so, however, with drawings where several lines led away from a single point" (Ellis, 1938, pp. 317–318).

Critics of Gelb and Goldstein, who examined Schn. many years later, found his tracing movements rather showy and theatrical, and doubted that the patient had a recognition impairment beyond such elementary visual problems as his constricted visual fields. For example, Bay (1953) and Jung (1949) noted that the patient was able to see and recognize most objects, and seemed to switch into his tracing routine only when performing tests for psychologists. It is possible that the patient had recovered in the more than twenty years that had elapsed since Gelb and Goldstein's studies. Indeed, the 40-year follow-up of Adler's patient HC (Sparr et al., 1991) also found the patient's real-life object and face recognition to have recovered considerably. However, she was still severely impaired in her perception of form per se, and sometimes used a tracing strategy when required to solve problems involving shape. This strategy had been in evidence when Adler (1944) first described this patient: "During the second week of her illness, the patient started to use her index finger to trace the contour of objects" (p. 244), and that even after considerable recovery, she would often "trace the contours of letters with her index finger in order to enforce perception" (p. 256). The fact that other patients, with similar visual impairments, have spontaneously adopted the same type of tracing strategy makes it unlikely that the tracing was purely an affectation to attract the interest of psychologists.

Landis et al. (1982) discuss the similarity of their case X to Gelb and Goldstein's Schn. in the spontaneous use of tracing strategies. They reported that "When allowed to trace, X could recognize simple geometric figures if the point of departure for tracing was unimportant (e.g., circle, triangle). With more complex figures he was misled by unimportant lines. He would give different answers for the same drawing, dependent upon the point of starting to trace, and often described incidental background features as meaningful. . . . Reading aloud was performed slowly but accurately. This 'reading' was accomplished by rapid tracing of letters, parts of letters or words with his left hand alone or with both hands. . . . [When] movement of the fingers could be prevented . . . this abolished reading." Also, like Gelb and Goldstein's case, X was "derailed" by slash lines, following them off of the figure being traced. Landis et al. provide another demonstration of what they call the "slavish" dependence on local continuity in their patient's tracing: when shown the stimulus in figure 2.4, the patient consistently read it as "7415."

Mr. S also spontaneously adopted a tracing strategy in a task in which he had to judge whether the orientation of two lines was the same or different. According to Efron (1968), "He carefully followed the contours of each by moving his head. Using this method, he frequently gave correct answers. However, when prevented from making head movements he could no longer perform the task" (p. 159). When asked to trace around a shape, Mr. S "will often go round a simple figure many times, not knowing that he has completed the task. . . ." In those cases in which he is asked to trace a complex object, he will almost always follow the contour of a single color area" (pp. 156–157). Finally, two of the cases were reported to have difficulty tracing figures by hand: Case ES (Alexander & Albert, 1983) had a general impairment in visually guided movements that precluded tracing, and RC (Campion, 1987) was reported to have difficulty tracing figures with hand movements. The latter case often resorted to

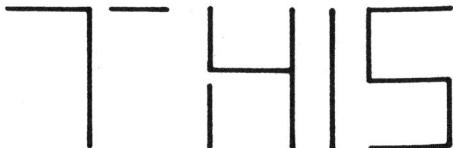

Figure 2.4
Patient X, studied by Landis et al. (1982), consistently read this stimulus as 7415.

spontaneous head movements when asked to identify an object, although it should be noted that Campion's interpretation was that RC seemed to be searching for the best view with these head movements.

Case DF displays a different form of visuomotor ability that has been the subject of intense study among neuropsychologists interested in perception and action. The earliest clue that DF had some degree of preserved visuomotor function came from observations of her reaching behavior. Whereas she could not accurately describe or compare the sizes, shapes, and orientations of objects, her motor interactions with the world seemed normal, including shaping her hand to the proper grip size while reaching to grasp a doorknob or a pencil. Milner, Goodale, and colleagues (Milner, Perrett, Johnston, Benson, Jordan, Heeley, Bettucci, Mortara, Mutani, Terazzi, & Davidson, 1991; Goodale, Milner, Jakobson, & Carey, 1991; Milner & Goodale, 1995) formalized this observation in a series of ingenious tests—for example, comparing DF's hand motions when asked to put a card through a slot, with the slot at different orientations, and when asked to describe the angle of the slot or to turn a second slot to match the angle of the first. Figure 2.5 shows the difference in accuracy between the two ways of accessing her perception of orientation: by conscious judgment or matching, and by action. The former is variable and inaccurate; the latter, flawless.

An interesting boundary condition on this dissociation was demonstrated by Goodale, Jakobson, Milner, Perrett, Benson, and Heitanen (1994), who repeated the slot experiment with a T-shaped opening. DF was unable to insert T-shaped blocks into the opening, suggesting that the preserved vision for action does not extend to full-blown shape perception.

How can this dissociation between DF's good visual motor abilities and poor explicit judgments of object shape and orientation be explained? Milner and Goodale suggest that the same dorsal visual pathways that have

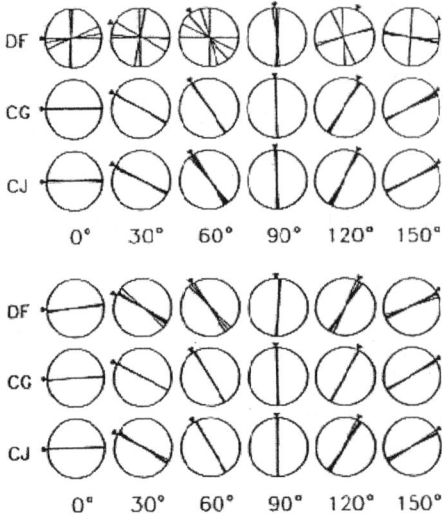

Figure 2.5
The performance of a visual form agnosic (DF) and control subjects at explicit judgments
of slot orientation (top) and at manipulating a card to fit through slots of the same orientations (bottom).

been hypothesized to underlie form-from-motion perception also mediate DF's visuomotor abilities. Specifically, they propose a functional disconnection between early visual representations in occipital cortex and
higher level representations of object appearance in the ventral stream.
Without access to ventral stream areas, DF cannot make explicit judgments of shape, size, and orientation. Her intact dorsal visual pathway is
nevertheless able to compute at least some of these properties for purposes
of action programming.

Shaun Vecera (2002) proposed an alternative hypothesis that builds
on the lower-level visual impairment that is evident in visual form agnosics. According to his account, the same degraded visual information
serves as input to both dorsal and ventral visual systems, but the dorsal visual system is more robust to degraded input than the ventral. He explains
this difference in robustness in terms of the complexity of the transformations that the stimulus representation must undergo between a retinotopic array and either shape or location representations; the transformation
to shape is more complex, and accordingly more fragile. Both the hy-

pothesized differences in complexity and their consequences for system robustness were confirmed by computer simulation. In either case, the dorsal pathway's independence of the ventral pathway in accomplishing visuomotor control is a feature of both explanations.

2.7   Neuropathology of Visual Form Agnosia

The neuropathology in these cases of visual form agnosia shows a fair degree of homogeneity. Five patients suffered carbon monoxide poisoning (Adler, 1944; Alexander & Albert, 1983; Benson & Greenberg, 1969; Campion & Latto, 1985; Milner et al., 1991), one suffered mercury poisoning (Landis et al., 1982), and one suffered a penetrating head wound (Gelb & Goldstein, 1918). Neurological signs, EEG, and structural imaging suggest that the brain damage in all of these patients was primarily posterior, affecting the occipital lobes and surrounding regions. With the exception of the penetrating head wound, the brain damage was diffuse and widespread rather than focal, and Bay (1953) suggested that the patient of Gelb and Goldstein was suffering less from the focal effects of his head wound than from increased intracranial pressure, which would also have diffuse and widespread effects. None of these cases has come to autopsy, and only HC underwent MRI scanning, which disclosed occipital atrophy. A CT scan of Campion's patient showed subcortical white matter lesions. Carbon monoxide is known to damage subcortical white matter and cortex diffusely (particularly the interlaminar connections between neurons), and to cause patchy, disseminated lesions. Landis et al. cite research showing that mercury poisoning affects the white matter of the occipital lobe.

Chapter 3

Dorsal Simultanagnosia

Some authors have classified the visual form agnosics just described with another group of patients who have a disorder known as simultanagnosia (e.g., Adler, 1944; Alexander & Albert, 1983; Bauer & Rubens, 1985; Luria, 1973). The term "simultanagnosia" was originally coined by Wolpert (1924) to describe a condition in which the patient accurately perceives the individual elements or details of a complex picture, but cannot appreciate its overall meaning. Patients with simultanagnosia resemble visual form agnosics in that they often have full visual fields, but may act as if they are blind. Furthermore, when presented with an array of stimuli, they often cannot identify stimuli indicated by an examiner. A final, qualitative similarity to visual form agnosics is that their perception has a "piecemeal" character to it: they may recognize some part or aspect of an object and guess the object's identity on the basis of the perceived feature. To further complicate things, simultanagnosia itself does not appear to be a homogeneous category. I have proposed that there are two distinct disorders that have been labeled "simultanagnosia" and often discussed interchangeably. To distinguish between them, I suggested the names "dorsal" and "ventral simultanagnosia," after their characteristic lesion sites (Farah, 1990).

3.1 Dorsal Simultanagnosia: A Case Description

Luria (1959, 1963) first associated Wolpert's rather general term with a specific type of perceptual deficit, in which only one object, or part of an object, can be seen at one time. This perceptual deficit is generally observed in the context of Balint's syndrome, which consists of (1) "psychic paralysis of gaze," an inability to direct voluntary eye movements to visual targets;

(2) optic ataxia, an inability to reach for or point to visual targets; and (3) a visual attentional deficit in which only one stimulus at a time is perceived, and even the attended stimulus may spontaneously slip from attention. The elements of the syndrome occasionally occur separately from one another (Coslett & Chatterjee, 2003; Rizzo, 1993), raising the possibility that they have different underlying mechanisms that are associated because of neuroanatomical proximity. It is the third element, termed simultanagnosia by Luria, that will be discussed here. Because the associated lesions are almost invariably bilateral parieto-occipital, affecting the dorsal but not the ventral visual pathway, I have called this "dorsal simultanagnosia."

A case described by Williams (1970) illustrates many of the prime features of dorsal simultanagnosia:

> A sixty-eight-year-old patient studied by the author had difficulty finding his way around because "he couldn't see properly." It was found that if two objects (e.g., pencils) were held in front of him at the same time, he could see only one of them, whether they were held side by side, one above the other, or one behind the other. Further testing showed that single stimuli representing objects or faces could be identified correctly and even recognized when shown again, whether simple or complex. . . . If stimuli included more than one object, one only would be identified at one time, though the other would sometimes "come into focus" as the first one went out. . . . If long sentences were presented, only the rightmost word could be read. . . . If a single word covered as large a visual area as a sentence which could not be read, the single word was read in its entirety. . . . If the patient was shown a page of drawings, the contents of which overlapped (i.e., objects were drawn on top of one another), he tended to pick out one and deny that he could see any others. (pp. 61–62)

3.2   General Characteristics of Dorsal Simultanagnosia

Dorsal simultanagnosia is not a common disorder, but over the decades a number of excellent case studies have been published. The earliest date from World War I, when bullets and shrapnel passing through soldiers' heads could, depending on the entry and exit points, cause the relatively symmetrical biparietal lesions of dorsal simultanagnosia (e.g., Holmes, 1918; Holmes & Horrax, 1919). More recent studies include those of Baylis, Driver, Baylis and Rafal (1994), Coslett and Saffran (1991), Gilchrist, Humphreys, and Riddoch (1996), Girotti, Milanese, Casazza,

Allegranza, Corridori, and Avanzini (1982), Godwin-Austen (1965), Hecaen and Angelergues (1954), Kase, Troncoso, Court, Tapia, and Mohr (1977), Luria (1959), Luria, Pravdina-Vinarskaya, and Yarbuss (1963), Tyler (1968), and Williams (1970). There is considerable similarity, from case to case, in the pattern of impaired and spared visual abilities.

The most striking feature of this syndrome is that although these patients are able to recognize most objects, they generally cannot see more than one at a time, and cannot shift rapidly from one to another. This is manifest in several ways: As with Williams's case, many cases can name only one of a set of objects. The description of complex scenes, which was Wolpert's defining criterion for simultanagnosia, is correspondingly slow and fragmentary. For example, the Cookie Theft picture in figure 3.1, which is a frequently used to assess the language abilities needed to describe a complex scene (Goodglass & Kaplan, 1978), can also be used to assess the relevant visual abilities. When viewing this picture, Coslett and Saffran's patient "identified the boy, girl and chair, but did not know who was standing on the chair or who was reaching for the cookie" (p. 1525).

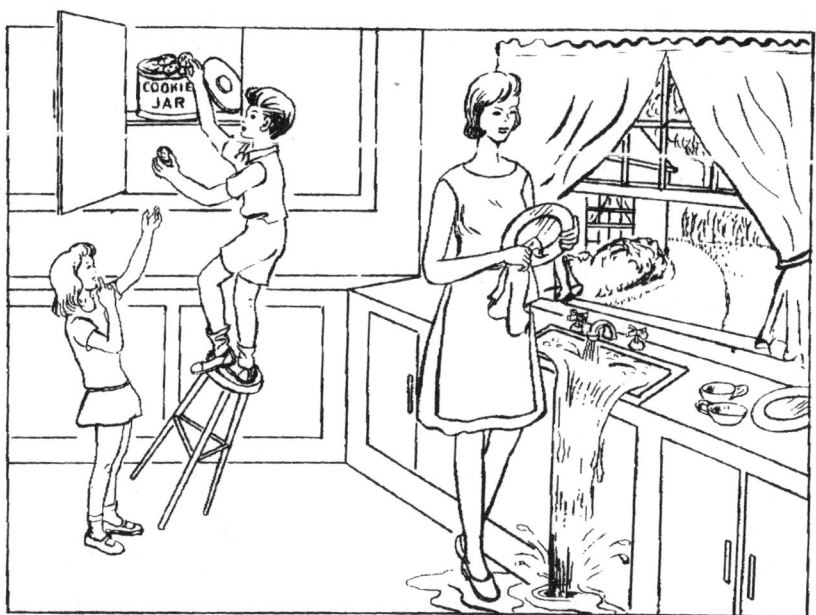

Figure 3.1
The Cookie Theft picture from the Boston Diagnostic Aphasia Examination.

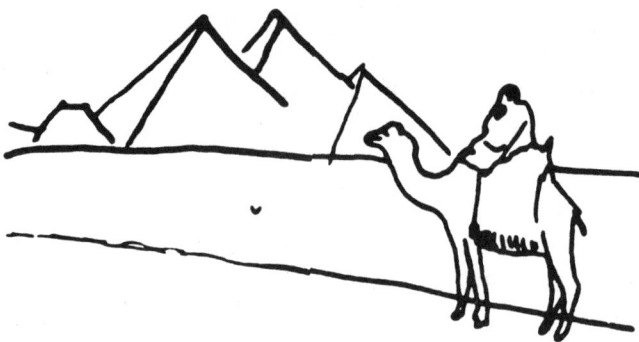

Figure 3.2
Drawing described by Tyler's (1968) patient, after prolonged scrutiny, as "a man looking at mountains." She never noticed the camel.

When shown the scene shown in figure 3.2 for 2 seconds, Tyler's subject said she saw "a mountain." When shown the figure for another 2 seconds, she said "a man," and did not indicate having seen the camel, desert, or pyramids, or realize that the man was related to what she had previously seen. When allowed over 30 seconds to look at the picture, she eventually said, "It's a man looking at the mountains." She said she never saw the "whole," but only bits of it that would "fade out" (p. 161). Similar complaints emerge in connection with reading: patients complain that words pop out from the page, then disappear and are replaced by other bits of text, not necessarily adjacent to the previous bit, making reading difficult or impossible.

Counting is another task that requires seeing more than one object at time, in order that the subject may keep track of which objects he has already counted and which he has yet to count. By contrasting visual counting ability with tactile or auditory counting ability, one can deduce whether or not the visual component of the task per se is the source of the patient's difficulty. Holmes (1918) describes the behavior of a typical case: "When asked to count a row of coins he became hopelessly confused, went from one end to the other and back again, and often passed over some of the series; but he succeeded in enumerating them correctly when he was allowed to run his left fingers over them" (p. 461).

These patients are often described as acting like blind people, groping for things as if in the dark, walking into furniture, and so on. For example, Coslett and Saffran say of their patient that "On one occasion she attempted to find her way to her bedroom by using a large lamp as a landmark; while walking toward the lamp she fell over her dining room table" (p. 1525). They add that she could find her way at home more easily with her eyes closed than with them open. This suggests that the problem is in fact quite different from the visual impairment of a blind person. Most authors have described the impairment as one of visual attention, for reasons stated succinctly by Holmes and Horrax (1919): "The essential feature was his inability to . . . take cognizance of two or more objects that threw their images on the seeing part of his retinae. As this occurred no matter on what parts of his retinae the images fell, it must be attributed to a special disturbance or limitation of attention, but visual attention only was affected as he did not behave similarly to tactile or other impressions" (p. 390). It follows from these observations that the attention system affected in these patients is not simply used for enhancing the processing of attended, relative to unattended, stimuli, but is necessary for the detection of stimuli.

There are some reports that even when dorsal simultanagnosics succeed in seeing an object, they will then "lose" it. This is particularly likely when the object is moving in a quick or unpredictable way, but can happen even with stationary objects (Godwin-Austen, 1965; Luria, 1959; Tyler, 1968). Rizzo and Hurtig (1987) studied the eye movements and subjective visual reports of three patients with dorsal simultanagnosia and found that in all three cases, stimuli seemed to disappear while under fixation. Thus, the stimulus disappearance in dorsal simultanagnosia is not secondary to eye movement problems. On the contrary, the tendency of these patients to make erratic, searching eye movements may sometimes be due to the spontaneous disappearance of the object they were viewing. This may reflect fatigue or habituation of central visual representations following the prolonged gaze that is characteristic of dorsal simultanagnosics, once their attention has locked onto an object.

3.3   Visual Disorientation

An additional characteristic of dorsal simultanagnosia is the inability to localize stimuli, *even when the stimuli are seen*. Because of this striking feature, the term "visual disorientation" is sometimes used as an alternative label for dorsal simultanagnosia. The ability to recognize a visible object without being able to localize it is one of the more surprising dissociations in neuropsychology, since it is so difficult for people without this disorder to imagine seeing and recognizing an object without knowing in which part of the visual field, or of space, they are seeing it. Yet this dissociation can be readily demonstrated in dorsal simultanagnosics, either by asking patients to point to or reach for the recognized visual stimulus or to describe its location. In its purest form it is specific to the visual modality, so that patients can locate auditory stimuli (Godwin-Austen, 1965; Holmes, 1918, case 3; Holmes & Horrax, 1919) or their own body parts when named (Holmes & Horrax, 1919; Kase et al., 1977, case 1) with great precision. Such patients provided the basis for early theorizing about the independence of spatial and object vision, now known to us through animal studies and imaging as the "two cortical visual systems" framework of Ungerleider and Mishkin (1982).

Are the visual disorientation, just described, and the attentional limitation of simultanagnosia one and the same underlying disorder, or are they merely associated because they depend on neighboring cortex? It seems likely that visual disorientation is secondary to, and an inevitable consequence of, the attentional disorder in dorsal simultanagnosia. This is because the location of an object can be specified only relative to another location, be it the subject's own body (in a pointing or reaching task), another object (when describing the object's location relative to another), or the origin of some abstract coordinate system. The inability of dorsal simultanagnosics to attend to two separate loci would therefore be expected to impair localization. A patient studied by Holmes (1918) supports this interpretation with his own introspections. When asked to describe the relative positions of two objects placed side by side, one above the other, or one nearer to him, the patient made many errors and spontaneously explained his performance by saying, "I can only look at one at a time" (p. 453).

The relation between representing visual location and attending to visual stimuli has been explored more fully explored in discussions of neglect (Chatterjee & Coslett, 2003). One research tradition explains neglect in terms of an impairment of attentional processing that affects the contralesional side of space (e.g., Posner et al., 1984), whereas another postulates an impaired internal representation of the contralesional side of space (e.g., Bisiach, Luzzatti, & Perani, 1979). However, it has been argued that these explanations are perfectly compatible, differing only in emphasis (Farah, 2000, chap. 8). Attention is not allocated to objects at locations in space, but rather to internal representations of objects at locations in space. Therefore, even according to an attentional account, neglect involves internal representations of the contralesional hemispace that cannot be used normally. Likewise, because attention operates on representations, a representational account of neglect implies that attention cannot be deployed in the contralesional hemispace. The same arguments apply to the bilateral impairment of location representation and attention in dorsal simultanagnosia.

3.4 Space-Based and Object-Based Attention

Cognitive psychologists distinguish between models in which visual attention is allocated to locations in space and to objects per se. Under most circumstances, these two alternatives are difficult to tell apart because every object has a location. With the appropriate experimental designs, however, it has been possible to tease the alternatives apart, and the evidence suggests that both forms of visual attention exist. Evidence for spatial attention includes demonstrations of that attention to one object will attentionally prime another object which either supersedes it in the same location (e.g., Posner, 1980) or occurs at a nearby location (e.g., Hoffman & Nelson, 1981). Evidence for object-based representations consist of demonstrations that two features can be attended to more effectively when they belong to the same object as opposed to different objects, even when the spatial distance between the features is held constant (Duncan, 1984) and is insensitive to the spatial distance between them (Vecera & Farah, 1994).

What is the nature of this attentional limitation in dorsal simultanagnosia? Is it a limitation on the region of visual space that can be attended to, or on the number of objects that can be attended to? The answer appears to be "some of both." The most salient limitation in dorsal simultanagnosia is on the number of objects that can be seen. Holmes and Horrax say of their patient, "It might be expected that as a result of this affection of visual attention he would be unable to see the whole of large objects presented to him at a near distance; but provided part of the image did not fall on the blind portions of his visual fields, this was never obvious on examination. He recognized objects and even complicated geometrical figures as promptly as normal persons. . . . He explained this by saying 'I seem to see the whole figure in the first glance', though occasionally he failed to do so if some peculiarity or prominent portion of it at once claimed his attention" (p. 390). Conversely, when attention is focused on a small object, even another small object nearby may not be seen. For example, Hecaen and Angelergues (1954, case 1) remark, "In lighting a cigarette, when the flame was offered to him an inch or two away from the cigarette held between his lips, he was unable to see the flame because his eyes were fixed on the cigarette" (p. 374). There is nevertheless some evidence that spatial factors play a role in the attentional bottleneck. On the rare occasions when multiple objects can be perceived, they are generally small, close together, and foveal (e.g., Holmes, 1918; Tyler, 1968).

The earliest experiments on object and spatial attentional limitations in dorsal simultanagnosia were carried out by Luria and colleagues. In one study (Luria et al., 1963) a patient was shown drawings of common objects at different sizes in a tachistoscope. He could name the objects presented one at a time, whether they subtended 6°–8° or 15°–20°. However, when two were shown simultaneously, even at the smaller size, the patient could only name one. Luria (1959) also reports that additional visual material could be perceived if grouped into a single object by so simple as change as connecting two forms with a line, as shown in figure 3.3. This observation has since replicated and extended by Godwin-Austen (1965) and Humphreys and Riddoch (1993).

The finding that the "fracture lines" of attentional impairment following bilateral dorsal visual system damage are influenced by the boundaries of objects might seem puzzling, given what we know about the division of labor between the dorsal and ventral visual systems. As already mentioned, there is abundant evidence supporting the division between "what," or object-related processing, and "where," or space-related processing. It is supposed to be the ventral visual system that represents objects, and the dorsal system that is concerned with spatial location.

The resolution of this conflict involves distinguishing between two types of object-based attentional effects, one of which is spatially mediated. This distinction is crucial to the interpretation of object-based at-

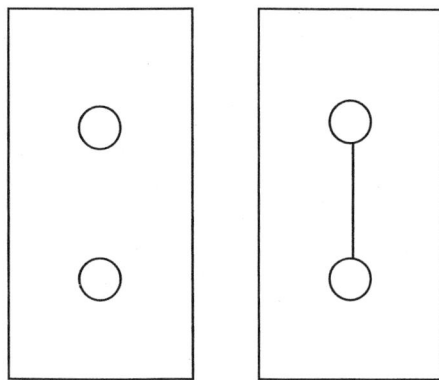

Figure 3.3
Stimuli of the type used by Luria (1959) and others to demonstrate the powerful effect of "objecthood" on the perception of shapes in dorsal simultanagnosia.

tention studies, in neglect as well as dorsal simultanagnosia, but has not always been clearly drawn (Buxbaum, Coslett, Montgomery, & Farah, 1996; Mozer, 2002). Spatially mediated object effects will emerge within any system that includes reciprocal activation between object representations and earlier, spatially formatted retinotopic representations. Consider the simple interactive model of spatial attention and object recognition shown in figure 3.4. The bidirectional arrows linking early retinotopic representations with the higher-level systems indicate the reciprocal nature of the influences between these pairs of systems. Spatial attention can select certain regions of the retinotopic array for further processing in either a "bottom-up" manner (i.e., a salient stimulus attracts attention) or a "top-down" manner (i.e., the person decides to shift attention to a certain region of the array). This is the most familiar mechanism by which attention is allocated to spatial locations. However, if the connection between the array and object representations enables top-down as well as bottom-up activation, then object knowledge will also influence the distribution of attentional activation of the array. Specifically, in addition to patterns in the array activating their corresponding object representations, those object representations will provide top-down support for their corresponding activation patterns in the array.

The process of object recognition therefore results in two types of activated object representation. The first is the object representation

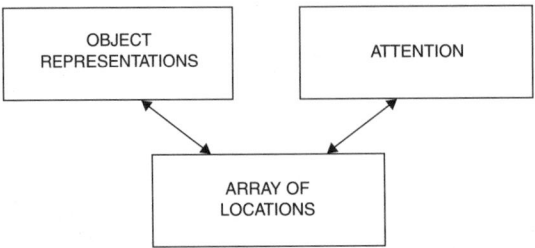

Figure 3.4
Model of the relations among the retinotopically formatted image representations of early and intermediate vision and two higher-level systems, visual object recognition and visual spatial attention. Each higher-level system receives input from the image, activating object representations and drawing attention to activated regions of the image. Each higher-level system also contributes activation to the image, in the form of top-down support for image features consistent with activated object representations and attentional activation in regions of the image to which attention has been drawn. The result of the visual object recognition pathway and the spatial attention pathway interacting in a common image representation is both the object effects in spatial attention observed with dorsal simultanagnosics and the spatial attentional effects on object recognition observed with ventral simultanagnosics.

proper, in the object system, which possesses various constancies such as shape and location constancy and is therefore not fundamentally a spatial representation. The second is the region of the retinotopic array containing the object image, activated by top-down influence from the first kind of object representation. In contrast to the distribution of attention by a purely spatial attentional "spotlight," which would be expected to activate simple ovoid clusters of array locations, the regions activated by object representations conform to the silhouette of the object in the array. Although such regions do, in a sense, represent object shape, the representation is fundamentally spatial, consisting of a set of locations or "pixels" in an array. Attention could in principle single out objects for further processing among the higher-level nonspatial representations of the object system, as Duncan (1984) suggested, or among the fundamentally spatial representations of the retinotopic array that have been shaped by top-down activation from the object system. In fact, both types of attention exist.

Vecera (1994) tested the predictions of the second type of account by showing that when an object is spatially attended, the attention tends to be distributed over the region of the image occupied by the object. Thus, a vertically oriented rectangle will attract spatial attention to regions above and below the rectangle's middle, and a horizontally oriented rectangle will attract spatial attention to the left and right. Using computer simulation, Mozer (2002) has shown that such a system of spatial attention can account for all of the demonstrations so far reported of object effects in the attentional limitations of parietal-damaged neglect patients. Figure 3.5 shows one such simulation.

Within this framework it is clear how the seemingly object-based limitation of attention in dorsal simultanagnosia can be accounted for in terms of damage to a fundamentally spatial attention system. Specifically, the impaired spatial attention system is operating on a spatial representation that has been parsed into objects by a normal object recognition system, and when it is unable to shift attention between regions, attention stays fixed on a single object's region, regardless of its size or complexity. This also explains the observation that although the visual attention of dorsal simultanagnosics is primarily limited to a single object, there is also some, relatively weaker, limitation on spatial extent.

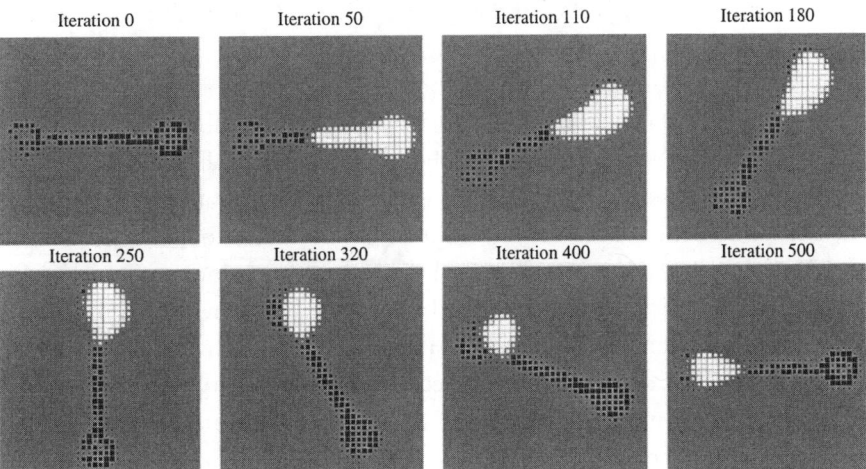

Figure 3.5
Computer simulation of the emergence of object-based attentional effects in a retino-topically formatted image representation (Mozer, 2002). Attention is initially allocated to the right end of the barbell, and tracks this portion of the object during rotation.

3.5   Spatial Relations Within and Between Objects

Objects and their parts are hierarchical, in that one can identify a bicycle as an object and a wheel as a part, or a wheel as an object and a spoke as a part. What, then, does it mean to say that attention is limited to one object at a time in dorsal simultanagnosia? Would it be limited to a bicycle, a wheel, or a spoke? The answer is that it depends. Just as we can see objects at various levels in a hierarchy, the damaged attentional system in dorsal simultanagnosia has flexibility in what it selects as an object, and both physical stimulus properties and higher cognitive processes contribute to this selection.

Luria (1959) asked a patient with dorsal simultanagnosia to describe two different versions of a Star of David. In the first version, the star was drawn all in the same color of ink. In the second, one of the two component triangles was drawn in red and the other was drawn in blue. The second version provided a stimulus in which there were two distinct "objects" or visual gestalts, the red and blue triangles, occupying roughly the same region of space and together occupying precisely the same region of space as the first version. When shown the first version, the patient consistently named the star. When shown the second version, the patient named either the red triangle or the blue triangle.

Dorsal simultanagnosics will sometimes appear to have an object recognition impairment because their visual attention will be captured by a part of the object to be recognized. For example, Tyler observed the following of his patient: "When shown a pitcher pouring water into a glass, she first noted the handle and said 'suitcase'. When asked to look again she spotted the glass, and remembering the handle she kept looking until she perceived the pitcher (now with the handle on it)" (Tyler, 1968, p. 158). This is reminiscent of Holmes and Horrax's comment that their patient sometimes failed to see a whole object if "some peculiarity or prominent portion of it at once claimed his attention." This attentional problem can interfere with recognizing objects. However, it is more accurate to say that it interferes with *seeing* objects, or seeing them at the "correct" level of the hierarchy of part-whole analysis; whatever dorsal simultanagnoscis can see, they can recognize. Furthermore, such problems are rare, since their attention is almost always claimed by what we would consider a single, whole object.

It is worth noting that the drawings of dorsal simultanagnosics are misleading as to their object perception. These patients are generally unable to copy drawings that they have recognized easily, and their attempts at copying have a characteristic "exploded" look, like the drawing of a bicycle shown in figure 3.6. This can be understood in terms of the necessity, in copying a picture, for drawing a part at a time, which requires patients to shift their attention to the individual parts of the shape and to position the parts with respect to each other. Of course, seeing multiple items and locating them with respect to each other is precisely what dorsal simultanagnosics cannot do. The patient whose copy is shown in figure 3.6 put it thus: "As soon as I lift my pencil from the paper I can't see what I have drawn and have to guess where to put the next detail" (Godwin-Austen, 1965, p. 455). Copying is not the straightforward test of shape perception that it might, at first glance, seem to be. This point will arise again in chapter 6, in the form of the opposite dissociation: good copies and impaired perception.

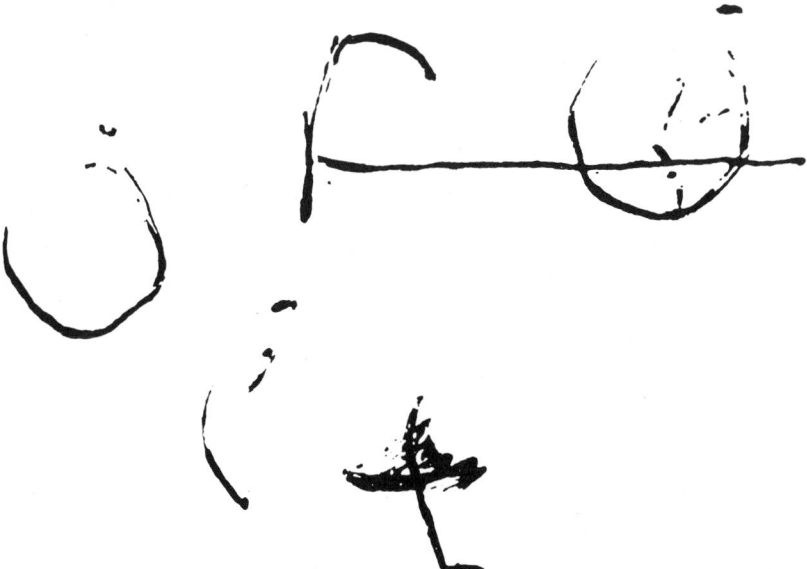

Figure 3.6
A drawing of a bicycle made by a dorsal simultanagnosic patient who was able to recognize objects and drawings, with the "exploded" look characteristic of such patients' copies.

"Objecthood" is not simply a matter of size or of visual complexity, as demonstrated by Luria (1959). When he showed a rectangle made up of six dots to a patient, the patient could see the rectangle, as well as recognize other geometric forms drawn with broken lines. However, as is the rule in dorsal simultanagnosia, counting was impossible, even counting the six dots of the rectangle he so easily identified. Apparently the patient could view the stimulus as dots, and therefore see a single dot at a time, or he could view it as a rectangle, and therefore see the entire rectangle. In the latter case, the patient was still unable to count the dots, presumably because once he started to count the dots, he would again be seeing them as dots and see only one at a time. In other words, the organization of the dots into a rectangle did not increase the patient's attentional capacity to more than one object; rather, it allowed the patient to view the set of dots as a single object. An implication of this is that the attentional system of dorsal simultanagnosics is sensitive to voluntary, "top-down" determinants of what constitutes an object.

The reading ability of dorsal simultanagnosics suggests that knowledge derived from previous learning also influences what our visual systems take to be an object. Recall Williams's (1970) observation that her patient could read a single word, regardless of whether it subtended a large or small visual angle, but a sentence subtending the same large visual angle could not be read. Other patients describe the experience of single words jumping out at them from a page (Girotti et al., 1982; Godwin-Austen, 1965; Luria, 1959; Luria et al., 1963; Hecaen & Angelergues, 1954, case 2; Holmes, 1918; Holmes & Horrax, 1919). The hypothesis that words function as objects in attracting attention was tested by Baylis, Driver, Baylis, and Rafal (1994) with a dorsal simultanagnosic patient. When shown letters in isolation, the patient recognized them easily, as would be expected, given that attention is limited to one object at a time. When shown four-letter words, he read them with high accuracy as well. On the other hand, his ability to name nonword strings of four letters was poor. Words and nonword strings do not differ in their objective visual complexity or wholeness, and thus provide compelling evidence for the role of knowledge in defining objects for the allocation of visual attention.

3.6   Neuropathology of Dorsal Simultanagnosia

The brain damage that causes dorsal simultanagnosia is bilateral and generally includes the parietal and superior occipital regions. In a few cases there has been evidence of damage confined to the occipital regions (Girotti et al., 1982; Rizzo & Hurtig, 1987), although in another only the superior parietal lobes were damaged (Kase et al., 1977, case 1). Etiologies likely to result in this configuration of damage, with preservation of ventral visual system areas, include the penetrating head injuries originally studied by Holmes (1918) and "watershed" infarction, in which a drop in blood pressure affects the most distal, or watershed, territory between the middle and posterior cerebral arteries. Middle cerebral artery strokes, although they commonly result in parietal damage, are not often the cause of dorsal simultanagnosia because of the need for bilateral lesions.

3.7   Visual Form Agnosia and Dorsal Simultanagnosia: Similarities and Differences

There is a "family resemblance" among several of the syndromes traditionally considered to be apperceptive agnosias. In the case of visual form agnosics and dorsal simultanagnosics, both may act effectively blind. They are unable to negotiate visual environments of any complexity, and will make random searching eye movements if asked to look at a particular object. Nevertheless, in both cases they may have relatively full visual fields and normal acuity and color perception. An additional similarity is that their perception appears to be piecemeal and confined to a local part or region of the visual field. Although visual form agnosics may seem generally more impaired at recognizing objects, both types of patients may evince object recognition difficulties and, when encountering these difficulties, both typically resort to guessing based on correct partial perceptions. Even the neuropathology fails to provide a clear basis for distinguishing among these patients. In both groups it is bilateral and posterior, and spares striate cortex to at least some degree, with cases of focal parieto-occipital damage occurring in both groups.

Despite these similarities, a closer look at the abilities and impairments of these groups of patients leads to the conclusion that the underlying deficits must be very different. Consider the "piecemeal" nature of perception in each case. In visual form agnosia only very local contour is perceived. It is so local that patients cannot trace across a break in a line, trace dotted lines, or avoid "derailment" onto irrelevant slashes drawn across a figure. This is not at all the case in dorsal simultanagnosia. Whole shapes are perceived, even if composed of dots or broken lines. What is piecemeal about the perception of dorsal simultanagnosics is the limitation of their vision to a single object or visual gestalt, without awareness of the presence or absence of other stimuli. Furthermore, in dorsal simultanagnosia the nature of the "piece" is at least partially determined by conscious attention (e.g., to the individual dots arranged in a rectangle or to the rectangle), whereas no such top-down influences have been noted to affect the piecemeal perception of apperceptive agnosics. The guessing strategies of visual form agnosics and dorsal simultanagnosics are likewise similar only on the surface. Although both make educated guesses about objects' identities based on partial perceptual information, the nature of the information used by each is different. Apperceptive agnosics use color, size, and texture, but do not use shape information. Dorsal simultanagnosics do use shape information. Furthermore, the shape perception of dorsal simultanagnosics is intact. A final difference is that whereas motion tends to facilitate shape perception by apperceptive agnosics, it interferes with perception by dorsal simultanagnosics.

Chapter 4

Ventral Simultanagnosia and Pure Alexia

There is another group of patients who have been called simultanagnosics, and who share the following characteristics with dorsal simultanagnosics. They are generally able to recognize a single object, but do poorly with more than one, and with complex pictures. Their introspections sound similar to those of dorsal simultanagnosics. For example, when viewing a complex picture, one patient said, "I can't see it all at once. It comes to me by casting my eye around" (Kinsbourne & Warrington, 1962, p. 466). As in dorsal simultanagnosia, reading is severely impaired. Furthermore, as in dorsal simultanagnosia, the size of the objects does not matter; the limitation is in the number of objects. It is therefore not surprising that the same label has been applied to these patients. However, on closer inspection these two groups of patients differ in important ways, implicating different underlying impairments. Ventral simultanagnosics are so called because the typical lesion is in the left temporo-occipital region.

Although ventral simultanagnosics cannot recognize multiple objects, they differ from dorsal simultanagnosics in that they can *see* multiple objects. This is evident in their ability to count scattered dots (Kinsbourne & Warrington, 1962), as well as in their ability to manipulate objects and walk around without bumping into obstacles. Furthermore, given sufficient time, they can recognize multiple objects. The one crucial activity of daily life that ventral simultanagnosics cannot perform is reading. The alexia of these individuals is so salient, compared to their other visual abnormalities, that they may be referred to simply as alexics. More specifically, their reading disorder is called "pure alexia" because it occurs in isolation from other visual and language disorders.

4.1   Ventral Simultanagnosia and Pure Alexia: A Case Description

A young man described by Warrington and Shallice (1980) exemplifies many of the characteristics of this syndrome. The individual was a 27-year-old deputy headmaster at a comprehensive school who five years earlier had suffered a brain hemorrhage and had undergone surgery to evacuate a left temporoparietal hematoma. His status when seen by the authors is described here.

At this time his only complaint was of being able to read only very slowly and haltingly, and of being unable to see words, especially long words, as a whole. . . . [He] was tested on the WAIS and obtained a verbal IQ of 125 and a performance IQ of 118. On both the Picture Arrangement and the Picture Completion subtests of the WAIS (the test stimuli are complex visual scenes) he obtained an age-scaled score of 13, which is within the high average range. . . . His perceptual skills appeared entirely normal; for example he scored 20/20 on a test of identifying objects from unconventional views (Warrington & Taylor, 1973). . . .

On the Schonell graded word reading test he scored at a high level, his performance being virtually error-free (98/100); on the Nelson reading test he obtained a reading IQ of 121 (42/50); his spelling was also entirely satisfactory. However, qualitatively, his reading was markedly abnormal. He was observed to spell out most words letter-by-letter either aloud or under his breath, and then reconstruct the word (correctly) from the auditory letter information. For example, he took thirty seconds to read the first fifteen words of a prose passage. Very short words appeared to be read relatively normally, but even these were read somewhat slowly. . . . He was able to read nonwords almost as efficiently as words. His mean time to read lists of 5 words and nonwords (the stimuli in both tests were 4 and 6 letters) was 13.3 and 14.0 seconds, respectively, and only very occasional errors were made. Numbers written in numerical form (for example 1,340,210) were read quickly and efficiently. There was no evidence of colour agnosia.

4.2   Ventral Simultanagnosia and Pure Alexia: Some Generalities

Pure alexia is more common than the other disorders discussed in this book. Perhaps because the syndrome is relatively familiar, recent articles tend to offer little in the way of patient description, such as performance on a variety of tests other than reading or real-life problems with reading, focusing instead on testing specific hypotheses. Earlier case reports, such as that of Warrington and Shallice excerpted above, are more generous with their background information on patients (see also Patterson & Kay, 1982; Warrington & Zangwill, 1957).

Of course, all reports document the letter-by-letter reading that is the hallmark of the syndrome. Even when patients do not spell words audibly, analysis of their single-word reading latencies as a function of number of letters in the word suggests a letter-by-letter strategy. Figure 4.1 shows the monotonic, almost perfectly linear, dependence of reading latency on word length in a pure alexic patient studied by Bub, Black, and Howell (1989). The negative acceleration of this function is probably attributable to the greater possibility of guessing the word before the last letters are read with longer words. Note the time scale on this figure: Even short words require several seconds for this patient, and each additional letter adds a second or more to the reading time. In summarizing the characteristics of seven pure alexic subjects from their research, Behrmann, Plaut, and Nelson (1998) noted a range in the time needed per letter, from 97 milliseconds for an extremely mild alexic to 1.4 seconds. Patients' reading rates can be considerably slower than that; I have seen pure alexics spend a minute or more on a word, although in such cases misidentifications of individual

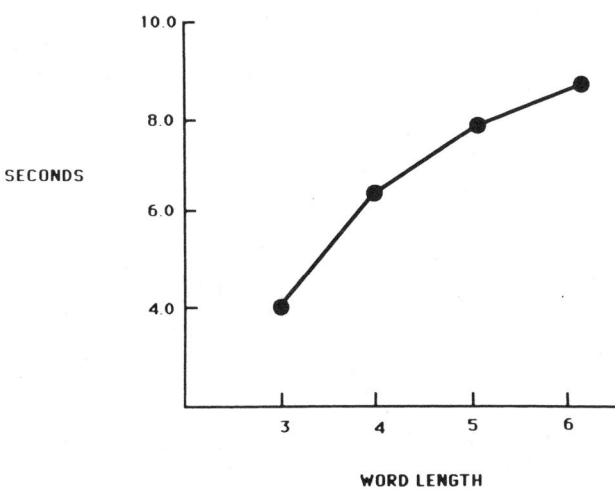

Figure 4.1
Single-word reading latency as a function of number of letters in the word for a pure alexic patient studied by Bub et al. (1989).

letters are also common. For that matter, however, it has been said that all pure alexics show some degree of impaired single-letter perception (Behrmann & Shallice, 1995).

In addition to the letter-by-letter reading strategy, the other general features of pure alexia concern visual and language ability. Patients' ability to understand spoken language and recognize objects is invariably tested and found to be grossly intact. When writing ability is tested, it also is intact, leading to the almost paradoxical finding of patients being unable to read what they themselves have written.

This form of alexia is called "pure" because other forms of visual pattern recognition appear preserved, as do spelling, writing, and other language-related abilities. However, a closer look at the visual abilities of these patients reveals a distinctive type of visual disorder, ventral simultanagnosia. Kinsbourne and Warrington (1962) first described the simultanagnosia of pure alexic patients. Their findings, and subsequent findings, are the focus of the next section.

4.3   Parallel Shape Recognition: A Dissociable Ability?

The nature of the perceptual impairment in ventral simultanagnosia was first investigated by Kinsbourne and Warrington (1962), with a series of elegant tachistoscopic experiments in which the speed of processing single and multiple visual shapes could be assessed. These experiments showed that the patients' tachistoscopic recognition thresholds for single forms (letters or simple pictures) were within normal limits, but that their thresholds departed dramatically from those of normal individuals when more than one form had to be recognized. Varying spatial factors, such as the size, position, and separation of the stimuli, had no effect; the visual processing "bottleneck" in these patients was determined solely by the number of separate forms to be recognized. Given that reading words involves the perception of multiple letters, this account of the visual impairment explains the alexia of these patients, and in particular the slow, letter-by-letter manner in which they attempt to read.

Levine and Calvanio (1978) replicated and extended the findings of Kinsbourne and Warrington with three new cases of what they termed "alexia-simultanagnosia." Among the novel results of their study were three findings that helped to pinpoint the locus of the processing impairment more precisely than Kinsbourne and Warrington's studies. First, Levine and Calvanio demonstrated that the difficulty with multiple stimuli is present even when the task does not involve naming the stimuli, but merely judging whether any two of the stimuli in an array are identical or not. This implies that the limitation is truly affecting perception per se, and not the process of labeling the percept. Second, subjects made more errors in this matching task when the letters in the display were visually similar (e.g., OCO, as opposed to OXO), again suggesting a visual locus for the processing breakdown. Finally, Levine and Calvanio contrasted the effects on subjects' performance of position cues presented just before and just after the stimulus array. If shape recognition per se is limited to just one item, then the pre-cue should improve performance because it allows the subject to recognize the one item that has been cued, but the post-cue should not, because it comes after the stimulus array has disappeared and thus cannot guide selective perception. In contrast, if the bottleneck is occurring after shape recognition, in some short-term memory buffer or labeling process, then the post-cues should also help. Levine and Calvanio found that subjects were helped by the pre-cues: if they knew in advance *which* letter (indicated by the position of a pre-cue) from a multi-letter array they were to report, they could do so accurately, even with the other letters present. However, if the cue came after perceptual processing had been completed, it did not help, again implicating visual recognition per se as the locus of impairment.

Why might the brain recognize multiple shapes with a distinct and separately lesionable system? Computationally, the recognition of multiple shapes poses a special problem, distinct from the problem of recognizing complex or unfamiliar shapes (to mention two other ways in which shape perception can be made difficult). The special problem for multishape recognition is cross talk, or interference, among the representations of separate shapes, which will be more severe the more distributed the representation.

Although distributed representation has many computational benefits and is used in a number of brain systems, including the visual object recognition system, it is not well suited to representing a number of items simultaneously. This is because once two distributed representations have been superimposed, it is difficult to know which parts of each of the two representations go together. This problem is illustrated in the top part of figure 4.2. The bottom part of figure 4.2 shows that one way around

Distributed Representation

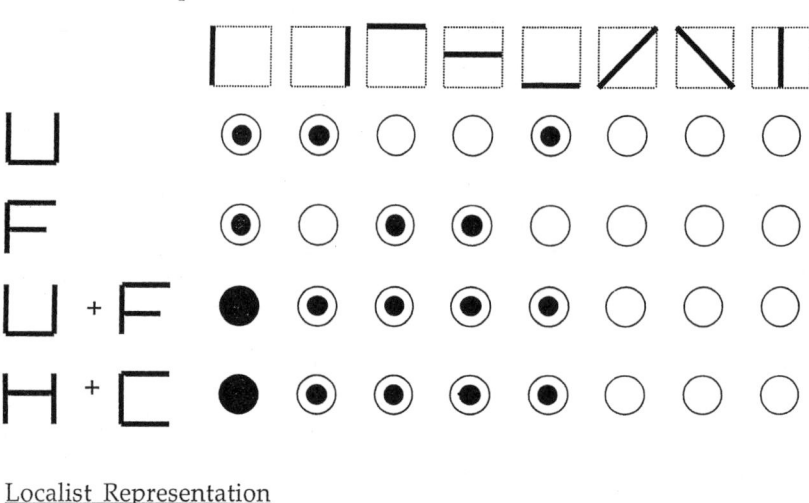

Localist Representation

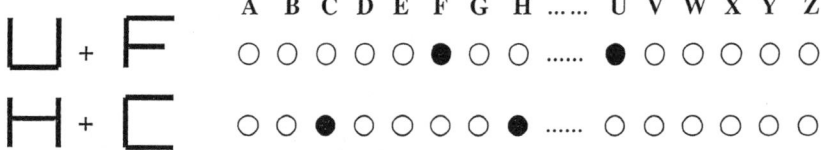

Figure 4.2
A demonstration of interference among multiple representations in distributed systems, and the lack of such interference in localist systems (from Farah, 2000).

this problem is to develop more localist representations. A tentative interpretation of the perceptual impairment of ventral simultanagnosics is that they have lost a region of cortex in which shape information is represented in a relatively more local manner.

4.4   *Are Ventral Simultanagnosia and Pure Alexia Equivalent?*

Although I have so far written as if pure alexia results from ventral simultanagnosia, this is not the only explanation that has been proposed for pure alexia. Indeed, in its simplest form—a general impairment in any kind of parallel shape recognition, which is noticeable only during reading—the explanation fails to account for certain observations, to be discussed. In this section the different types of explanation for pure alexia will be reviewed, along with the evidence for and against each.

The *disconnection account* of pure alexia was proposed by Dejerine (1892), and more recently championed by Geschwind (1965). According to this account, reading consists of associating visual information in occipital cortex with language representations in posterior language areas. This is done by way of the left angular gyrus, adjacent to Wernicke's area, which is hypothesized to contain stored multimodal associations linking the visual and sound patterns of printed words. Thus, pure alexia results from any lesion that disconnects the visual cortex from the left angular gyrus. The neuropathology of pure alexia is generally consistent with this hypothesis (e.g., Damasio & Damasio, 1983; Greenblatt, 1983), often involving a left occipital lesion (causing blindness in the right visual field) and damage to the adjacent splenium (disconnecting left visual field information from the left hemisphere). Despite the anatomical support for this interpretation of pure alexia, it is not an altogether satisfying explanation. For one thing, although it is not in any way *inconsistent* with the letter-by-letter reading strategy of pure alexic patients, it also is not *explanatory* of this highly characteristic feature of the syndrome.

It is, of course, possible that disconnection may contribute to some particularly severe cases of pure alexia. I recall one patient who was virtually unable to read at all, and whose letter-by-letter reading often involved letters that bore no relation to the word he was looking at. His oral verbal responses seemed to be running free, independent of visual input, with a tendency toward perseveration, and his picture naming had the same unrelated and often perseverative qualities. The total impression was of exactly a disconnection in the pathways that normally link visual input and verbal output. Yamadori (1980) reported two relatively severe cases of pure alexia with what he called "unilateral dyscopia," the inability to copy written characters with one hand. In both cases the right-hand copies were worse than the left-hand, consistent with the inability of visual information to reach the left hemisphere. The more severe case, who was entirely unable to read written characters, showed the more complete dissociation in copying between the left and right hands.

The *ventral simultanagnosia* account was the next to be proposed, by Kinsbourne and Warrington in 1962 and more recently advocated by Marcie Wallace and myself (Farah & Wallace, 1991). In the research already summarized in section 4.3, pure alexic patients were shown to have an impairment in the rapid recognition of multiple shapes using tachistoscopic methods. This impairment can also be demonstrated with more natural stimulus presentations. Wallace and I administered simple paper-and-pencil tasks that stress the rapid encoding of multiple visual shapes to a pure alexic, and found a severe impairment, a finding that has since been replicated by Sekuler and Behrmann (1997) in three additional patients.

So far the support for the ventral simultanagnosia account has taken the form of associations between impairments in multiple parallel shape recognition and letter-by-letter reading. Evidence from associations is subject to a particular type of alternative explanation, specifically that there are two separate abilities which depend on neighboring brain regions and which are therefore likely to be spared or impaired together. The ambiguity of associational data provided the motivation for us to manipulate the difficulty of visual perception and assess its effect on the reading of a pure alexic (Farah & Wallace, 1991). We used additive factors logic to identify the stage of reading that gives rise to the abnormal word length effect (i.e., the stage of reading at which the process is forced to proceed letter by letter), and specifically to test whether it is the visual shape recognition stage of processing. According to additive factors logic, if two experimental manipulations affect the same stage of processing, their effects will be interactive, whereas if they affect separate stages, their effects will be additive (Sternberg, 1969).

We presented a pure alexic with words of varying length to read, printed either clearly or with spurious line segments superimposed, as shown in figure 4.3. This manipulation of visual quality would be expected to affect the stage of visual shape recognition. We found that word length and visual quality interacted in determining reading latency. Specifically, the word length effect was exacerbated by visual noise, as shown in figure 4.4. This finding is consistent with a visual shape recognition locus for the word length effect in this experiment, and, in more general terms, with the hypothesis that an impairment in the rapid perception of multiple shapes underlies pure alexia. Unfortunately, the most straight-

point
moral
until

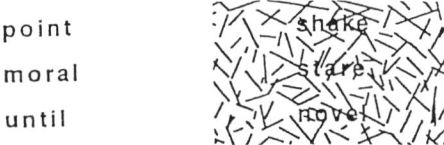

Figure 4.3
Examples of normal and degraded word stimuli used in a study of pure alexia.

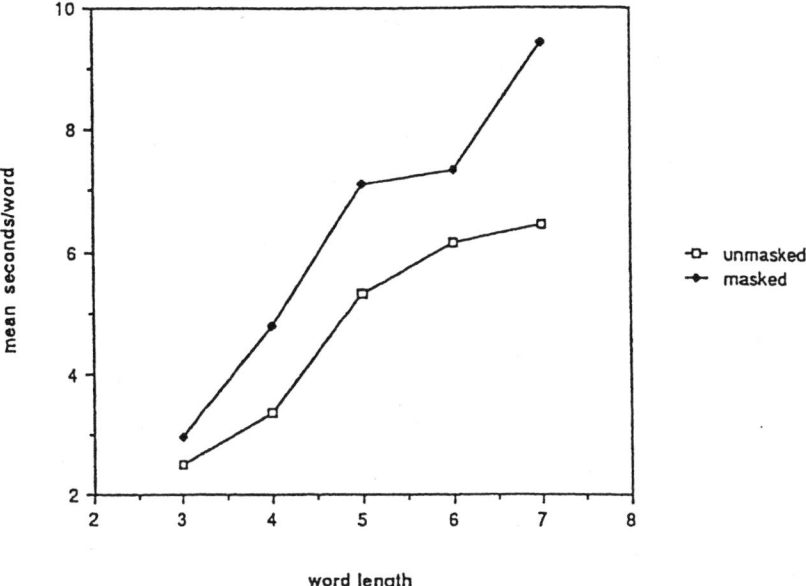

Figure 4.4
The interaction of visual degradation by masking and the word length in a pure alexic patient.

forward version of the ventral simultanagnosia account does not explain the observation that number recognition is preserved in some pure alexic patients, as it was in Warrington and Shallice's (1980) case. It also fails to explain why single letters are often misperceived in pure alexia.

The third major approach to explaining pure alexia is as an *orthography-specific impairment*. There are a number of levels of orthographic representation that could be impaired in pure alexia, from individual letters to whole word representations. Warrington and Shallice (1980) proposed that pure alexia was the result of damage to relatively high-level orthographic representations of words and morphemes. They called these representations "word forms" and pointed out that a loss of word forms could explain the characteristic letter-by-letter reading of pure alexics, since their visual word recognition cannot make use of word forms, and therefore must proceed via individual letter recognition and knowledge of spelling.

The evidence presented by Warrington and Shallice in favor of their hypothesis was of two kinds. First, they assessed various visual capabilities in an attempt to rule out visual perception as the locus of impairment. By a process of elimination, this would strengthen the case for a word form impairment. However, despite having used a number of different perceptual tasks, many of which involved displays of multiple items, none of the tasks specifically taxed the process of rapid perception of multiple shapes, which is the leading alternative hypothesis. For example, some of the tasks were not speeded, some involved foreknowledge of target locations (eliminating the need to recognize all but the target stimuli), and so on (see Farah & Wallace, 1991, for a detailed review of these tasks).

Second, Warrington and Shallice manipulated reading difficulty in two ways that they believed would render subjects relatively more dependent on visual word forms. In one experiment they compared the reading of print to the reading of script, and found performance with script to be worse. In a second experiment they compared reading words that had been presented tachistoscopically, for half a second, to reading nontachistoscopic word presentations, and found a marked decrement in reading performance with tachistoscopic presentations. Although these manipulations could well increase the reader's reliance on word forms, they would also make reading harder for a ventral simultanagnosic, and therefore do not discriminate between the accounts.

The word form hypothesis has not fared well in the face of more recent demonstrations that at least some pure alexic subjects show a "word superiority effect." The word superiority effect refers to the facilitation of letter perception when letters occur in the context of a word or pseudoword, relative to a nonword or, in some cases, no flanking letters at all (Reicher, 1969; Wheeler, 1970). The facilitation of letter perception by word or wordlike contexts is not simply the result of a bias to guess letters that would make a word, because it is observed even in forced-choice tasks when both choices make a word: for example, when the stimulus is ROAD and subjects are asked whether the second character is an O or an E.

The word superiority effect might seem paradoxical at first, for one usually thinks of letters being perceived before words, yet here words are influencing letter perception. The key to understanding this effect is to note that while letters are indeed perceived before words, in the sense that their representations begin to be activated before word representations begin to be activated (Johnston & McClelland, 1980), letter activation may not be complete by the point at which word representations begin to be activated. Assuming that activated words feed activation back down to their component letter representations, as well as compete with one another in a winner-take-all manner, then words, most likely on the basis of midprocess letter recognition, will reinforce perception of those letters. An early and influential connectionst model, by McClelland and Rumelhart (1981), demonstrates the way in which such within-level competitive interactions and between-level reinforcing interactions together account for most of the findings concerning word superiority in letter perception. Figure 4.5 shows a schematic depiction of part of their model.

The word form hypothesis predicts an absent or at least attenuated word superiority effect in pure alexic subjects. However, a number of pure alexic patients have shown word superiority effects, in some cases comparable to control subjects' (see Behrmann, Plaut, & Nelson, 1998, for a review), leaving the word form hypothesis with little supporting evidence and substantial disconfirming evidence.

A final account of pure alexia is a hybrid of the preceding two that involves *specialization within specialization* in the brain. One specialization is for the rapid or parallel encoding of multiple shapes, which I earlier argued could be accomplished by developing more localist representations. According to this account, the general manifestations of ventral simultanagnosia result from damage to such an area. However, a further specialization within this area can be hypothesized to occur for letter and word representation because these are the stimuli most frequently processed in this area. The development of the latter specialization has been shown to emerge naturally from basic principles of neural computation.

Thad Polk and I have explored some of the ways in which neural networks respond to statistical regularities in our visual environment, particularly orthographic regularities, using a "self-organizing system," a network that learns without an external source of information conveying "right" or "wrong." Indeed, in such systems there is no "right" or "wrong" because there is no target pattern to be learned. Rather, the strength of connections among the neuronlike units of such a network is changed simply as a function of the correlations among the activity levels of the units in the network. The best-known learning rule for self-organizing systems is the Hebbian rule: "Neurons that fire together wire together." In other words, when the activity levels of two units are positively correlated, the connection strength between them increases. This increases the likelihood that their activations will be correlated in the future, since activation of

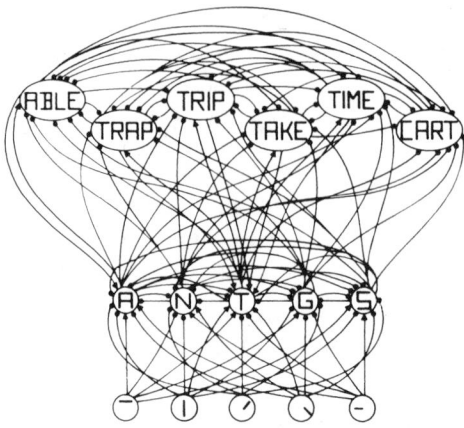

Figure 4.5

Illustration of the interactive activation model of word recognition. Letter units are initially activated by an amount proportional to the input they receive from the units representing their constituent features. The letter units then pass activation on to the words with which they are consistent. For example, if there appears to be a "t" in the first position, that will cause the words "trap," "trip," "take," and "time" to gain activation. In addition, word units are inhibited by the activation of units that are inconsistent with the word. For example, "able" will be inhibited by the unit representing an initial "t," since activation in these units represents incompatible hypotheses, and "able" will also be inhibited by activation in other word units for the same reason. So far, this model would seem to account for word recognition, but it is not yet clear how it accounts for the word superiority effect, nor is it clear how it accounts for phenomena involving pseudowords, that is, statistical approximations to real words. The word superiority effect is explained by postulating feedback from the word level to the letter level. Switching to a set of examples different from those shown in figure 4.5, if the word shown is "read," and perception of the letter in the second position is just barely adequate, so that the "e" unit is ever so slightly more activated than the "o" unit, then this will give the edge to the word "read" over the word "road." Interword inhibition will then drive the activation of the "road" unit down, and feedback from the word level to the letter level will therefore consist of greater "top-down" support for "e" than for "o." Thus, people will be more accurate at discriminating "e" from "o" in the context of "read" than in a nonword context or alone. Why should pseudowords also give rise to superior letter perception, given that there are no units corresponding to them at the word level? Because pseudowords are sufficiently similar to real words that their constituent letters will at least partially activate some real word units. "Yead," for example, will activate "year," "bead," read," and so on. Once these word units have become activated, they will inhibit other word units that are less consistent with the activated letter-level units, and will provide top-down support for the letters that do occur in the words similar to "yead," including, for example, the "e" in the second position.

one will cause the other to become active by virtue of the strengthened connection. In this way, the network develops a repetoire of stable patterns of activation, in the sense that activation patterns which are close to the learned pattern (e.g., contain part of it) will be transformed into the learned pattern and tend to remain active. These stable patterns can be viewed as representations of whatever inputs to the network evoke the patterns.

If it is assumed that prior to learning, neighboring neurons have excitatory connections among them, such that activating one neuron tends to activate its neighbors, then it is possible to account for a number of aspects of cortical representation by the simple mechanism of Hebbian learning. For example, topographic maps such as the somatosensory homunculus arise because neighboring locations in the input to be represented (locations on the body surface, in the case of the homunculus) tend to be activated at the same time. Because of the short-range excitatory connections, this biases neighboring units of the network to represent neighboring regions of the input (e.g., Merzenich, 1987).

In the foregoing examples, statistical regularities in the environment interact with correlation-driven learning to give rise to organized cortical representations. For example, the statistical regularity of correlated activity at neighboring locations of the input space leads to topographic mapping of that space. Polk and I reasoned that orthographic statistical regularities in the visual environment would also interact with the correlation-driven learning of self-organizing systems in much the same way. The most obvious aspect of the statistics of orthography is the co-occurrence among letters. If you are looking at one letter, you are probably seeing many other letters, and you are unlikely to be seeing a digit. In contrast, if you are looking at a digit, there is a good chance that you are seeing other digits at the same time, rather than letters.

We found that, across a number of variations in simple Hebbian-type learning rules and network architectures, the co-occurrence of letters with letters and digits with digits led the network to segregate its letter and digit representations (Polk & Farah, 1995a). In other words, the network developed specialized letter and digit areas. This is because once a unit in the network has begun to represent one letter, spreading activation will cause its neighbors to become active when that letter is presented. Other items that are presented along with that letter will therefore be biased to come to be represented by the neighbors of the original letter's representing unit, because those neighbors will be active during the presentation of the other item. The fact that the co-occurring items will usually be other letters means that other letters' representations will cluster around that first one.

If the statistics of the input are adjusted to take into account the greater co-occurrence of letters with letters than of numbers with numbers, the simulation then tends to organize with letter areas only. Digits and other shapes remain intermixed. This accounts for the observation that letter perception may be worse than digit perception in some pure alexic subjects.

The idea that co-occurrence drives the organization of visual shape representations toward a segregated letter area was tested with a group of subjects whose visual experience with letters and digits conforms to very different statistics. Thad Polk and I tested postal workers who spend eight hours on alternate days sorting Canadian mail by postal code. These codes consist of alternating letters and numbers, for example, M5M 2W9. As a measure of the segregation of letter representations from number representations, we used the degree to which letters pop out, in a visual search task, against a background of numbers. If letter representations are indeed segregated from number representations, then the presence of a letter can be detected by the presence of activity in the letter area, without the need to individually recognize the characters in a display. Letters are indeed detected among numbers faster than among letters (e.g., Jonides & Gleitman, 1972), consistent with the existence of segregated letter representations in normal subjects. As predicted, Canadian mail sorters showed less of a difference between these two conditions than postal worker control subjects (Polk & Farah, 1995b). A variation on the same type of mechanisms can also create case-invariant letter representations, sometimes referred to as abstract letter identities (Polk & Farah, 1997). In light of this, it is interesting to note that pure alexic subjects are generally disproportionately impaired in visual matching tasks requiring cross-case matching (Behrmann & Shallice, 1995; Bub, Black, & Howell, 1989; Kay & Hanley, 1991; Reuter-Lorenz & Brunn, 1990).

If letter representations are segregated within the visual system, by the type of mechanism proposed here, then our visual system does contain orthography-specific components and pure alexia could follow from damage to such a component. However, because this component segregates out within an area that is already specialized for representing multiple shapes simultaneously, most lesions would be expected to result in some degree of general impairment in the recognition of multiple shapes as well as a more severe impairment for the recognition of orthography, and an especially severe impairment for tasks requiring the representation of abstract letter identity, such as cross-case matching.

Much of the research on pure alexia since the 1990s has focused on a binary decision: Is it a visual impairment affecting all types of stimuli, or is it orthography-specific? Reluctantly, I have come to the conclusion that the truth is probably more complex than either of these two alternatives. Although I was initially impressed with the evidence for a visual impairment that extends beyond orthography, an accumulation of clinical observations suggests that visual letter perception, if not word perception, may be disproportionately impaired in some pure alexics. Both observations can be accommodated by a hypothesis of "specialization within specialization." The more general visual impairments are caused by damage to a brain region specialized for rapid encoding of multiple shapes, which may involve a computational strategy of localist representation. Among the shapes most frequently processed in this area are letters, seen mainly in the context of words and by the mechanisms proposed by Polk and myself (Polk & Farah, 1995a; 1997); these will segregate out within this multiple shape-encoding area, forming an even more specialized subarea, and possibly coming to represent abstract letter identities. Depending upon the exact location of the lesion relative to these areas, pure alexics would be expected to have a visual impairment for rapid encoding of multiple visual shapes, with varying degrees of orthography-specificity.

4.5 Dorsal and Ventral Simultanagnosia: Similarities and Differences

Ventral simultanagnosics share a number of characteristics with the patients discussed in the previous chapter. Like dorsal simultanagnosics, they perceive complex visual stimuli in a piecemeal manner, and both types of patients have great difficulty reading. Also like dorsal simultanagnosics, the limitation on what they perceive is not determined by size or position but by number of objects. As a result, the two types of disorder were discussed interchangeably for many years; indeed, they were both simply referred to as simultanagnosia.

Despite these similarities, a closer look at the abilities and impairments of these groups of patients leads to the conclusion that the underlying deficits must be very different. In dorsal simultanagnosia, perception is piecemeal in that it is limited to a single object or visual gestalt, without awareness of the presence or absence of other stimuli. In ventral simultanagnosia, *recognition* is piecemeal, that is, limited to one object at a time, although, in contrast to dorsal simultanagnosia, other objects are *seen*.

4.6   Neuropathology of Ventral Simultanagnosia and Pure Alexia

The lesions responsible for ventral simultanagnosia and pure alexia affect the left posterior temporal or temporo-occipital cortex, and the disorder has been considered a localizing sign for damage there (Kinsbourne & Warrington, 1963). This localization accords well with the results of functional neuroimaging studies, which show selective activations within this zone (Petersen, Fox, Snyder, & Raichle, 1990; Polk & Farah, 2001; Price, Wise, Watson, Patterson, Howard, & Frackowiack, 1994). The precise location of orthography-specific activation varies somewhat from imaging study to imaging study, perhaps as a result of different materials and experimental designs.

Chapter 5

Perceptual Categorization Deficit and Disorders of Orientation Processing

The patients in the foregoing chapters have clinically evident problems, and much of what is known about them comes from clinical case descriptions. There are other patients who have been termed "visual agnosic" but whose disorders rarely cause them problems in everyday life. These types of agnosia are demonstrated in experimental tasks, and may be studied in groups of patients delineated by lesion site as well as in individual cases selected for their poor performance on the relevant tests.

In addition to their subtlety, the disorders of this chapter have another feature in common: they are detected using misoriented stimuli and are presumed relevant to orientation constancy in object recognition. Orientation constancy is our ability to perceive an object's shape as constant across changes in the object's orientation relative to us. It is at the heart of the problem of object recognition, since the retinal image with which object recognition begins can change drastically as the object rotates. This is particularly true of rotations in depth (i.e., out of the picture plane) because of foreshortening and occlusion.

Approaches to achieving orientation constancy are of two general types: either transform the perceived image into a format that is orientation-invariant, such that two different views of a shape map to the same orientation-invariant representation, or maintain the image format and apply normalizing transformations to bring the different images of a shape into alignment. In the first category are the use of orientation-invariant features and object-centered representations and in the second is mental rotation (see Farah, 2000, chap. 3, for more discussion of these alternatives). Which approach or approaches are taken by the human visual system is an open question.

5.1   Perceptual Categorization Deficit

De Renzi, Scotti, and Spinnler (1969) first described this disorder, whose main feature is difficulty matching three-dimensional objects across shifts of perspective. In their study, the objects being matched were faces, and the poorest performance on this task was found in right hemisphere-damaged patients with visual field defects, implying that the critical lesions were in the posterior right hemisphere. This initial work was followed by a series of well-known studies by Warrington and her colleagues, who somewhat confusingly refer to the disorder as "apperceptive agnosia." Warrington and Taylor (1973) showed that right posteriorly damaged patients were no worse than normal subjects at naming objects photographed from conventional views like that shown in figure 5.1a, but were, on average, quite poor at naming the same objects photographed from unconventional views like that shown in figure 5.1b. Warrington and Taylor (1978) found that even when patients had recognized the conventional view, they were sometimes unable to see that the corresponding unconventional view was the same object in a matching task. The critical lesion site for this impairment, based on superimposed reconstructions of lesions in Warrington and Taylor's (1973) study, appears to be the right posterior inferior parietal lobe.

In addition to the group studies just described, in which a large number of brain-damaged patients are grouped by hemisphere or quadrant of damage and some summary measure of the performance of these anatomically defined groups is compared with the performance of control subjects, there have also been case studies of perceptual categorization deficit. Warrington and James (1988) present three such cases. Right posteriorly damaged patients performed within normal limits on tests of elementary visual function, including the Efron (1968) rectangle matching task (figure 2.2), but performed extremely poorly on a series of tests of perceptual categorization. They were able to recognize only six to eight out of twenty unconventional views of objects, like the photograph in figure 5.1b, although they named almost all of the same objects (seventeen to twenty out of twenty) when shown them later from conventional perspectives, like the photograph in figure 5.1a. When asked to name silhouettes of objects in an unconventional foreshortened orientation, and when shown the silhouettes of objects being rotated from unconventional to conventional

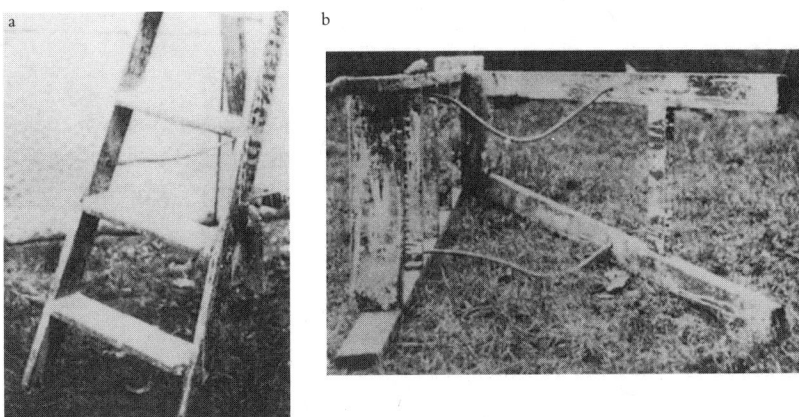

Figure 5.1
Usual and unusual views, from the research of Warrington and colleagues (e.g., 1985).

perspectives, they made many errors and required that the object be rotated to a more conventional perspective before being able to identify it.

5.2   Perceptual Categorization Deficit: Characterizing the Underlying Impairment

On the face of things, perceptual categorization deficit appears to correspond neatly to a loss of orientation constancy. For this reason patients with an apparently selective impairment of this ability were of great interest. Indeed, Warrington's research on perceptual categorization deficit was the only neuropsychological evidence cited by David Marr in his landmark book on vision (1982). He interpreted it as an inability to transform the image representation to an object-centered representation of shape, from which perspective and other aspects of the viewing conditions had been eliminated

There are a number of reasons to question the relevance of perceptual categorization deficit to understanding visual object recognition, and even orientation constancy in particular. Warrington (1985) points out that orientation shifts are not the only manipulations of perceptual quality that pose problems for these patients. She cites unpublished data of Warrington and Ackroyd demonstrating that the matching impairment extends to photographs of objects with uneven lighting—for example, the

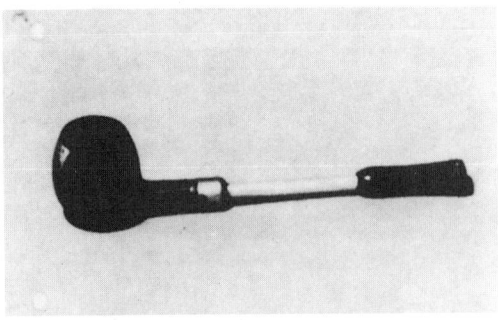

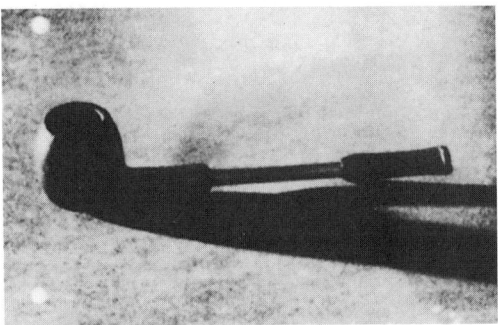

Figure 5.2
Usual and unusual lighting, from the research of Warrington and colleagues (e.g., 1985).

pair of pictures shown in figure 5.2. Warrington therefore describes the impairment in a fairly general way, as a failure of "perceptual categorization," rather than a failure of orientation constancy, suggesting that patients can no longer categorize perceptually dissimilar images in terms of the distal stimulus object that they have in common. However, even this more general interpretation meets with difficulties, as Warrington herself later noted.

One problem is that these patients are generally not impaired in everyday life. Their deficit is manifest only on specially designed tests. This is not what one would expect if so fundamental an object recognition process were impaired. A second and related problem is that these patients have not, in fact, been demonstrated to have an impairment in matching objects across different views. What, you say? Isn't this the impairment for which this group of patients is known? Although perceptual categorization deficit involves a problem in matching different views of objects, all that has been demonstrated for familiar real objects is a problem matching a usual to an *unusual* view. Although one could construct a test in which different usual views of objects must be matched, the tests used so far have always included an unusual view.

The way we recognize all manner of usual object views is swift and automatic; seeing and recognizing feel simultaneous, and metaphors of "visual inference" are just that. In contrast, when people recognize unusual views, the process is protracted, often requiring several seconds, and does sometimes involve conscious inference. Data from control subjects in these studies of unusual view recognition shows a low but nonzero error rate (e.g., Warrington & Taylor, 1973). It is therefore likely that the recognition or matching of unusual views requires a kind of effortful processing above and beyond object perception proper. Such processing might more aptly be called visual problem-solving than visual recognition.

When the quality of visual input is degraded, as it generally is following right parietal lesions, patients may find the problems unsolvable. Support for such an interpretation comes from Mulder, Bouma, and Ansink (1995), who administered a range of perceptual categorization tasks to patients whose visual sensory and attentional abilities had been assessed. They found a strong association between perceptual categorization, on the one hand, and sensory and attentional function on the other. Although two patients with left neglect performed within normal limits on the perceptual categorization tasks, the authors point out that such patients were administered the perceptual categorization tests in a way that minimized the effects of neglect.

In sum, as simple and informative as perceptual categorization deficit first appeared to be, in the end it has not shed much light on visual object recognition. Indeed, following an unfortunate pattern seen many times before in psychology (e.g., the lexical decision task and the P300), the effort to understand perceptual categorization deficit in all its unexpected complexity may have superseded the effort to use it to understand more basic questions about mind and brain.

5.3   Orientation Agnosia

If perceptual categorization deficit is not evidence for a dissociable system of orientation-invariant object vision, are there other neuropsychological syndromes that are? One possible candidate is a disorder that Turnbull and colleagues have named "orientation agnosia," described in a small number of right hemisphere-damaged patients (Turnbull, Laws, & McCarthy, 1995; Turnbull, Carey, & McCarthy, 1997; Turnbull, Beschin, & Della Sala, 1997). Patients with orientation agnosia are able to recognize drawings of objects that have been rotated in the picture plane, but are impaired at recognizing the pictures' orientation. For example, given a drawing of bus, one patient correctly named it but oriented the picture upside-down. The orientation errors are manifest when patients select the orientation for a picture, when they attempt to match pictures, and when they copy pictures. Figure 5.3 shows copies of three geometric patterns made by an orientation agnosic.

The first of the two approaches to object constancy described earlier, the use of orientation-invariant shape representations, suggests a tantalizing interpretation of this disorder: it results from preserved orientation-invariant representations, unaccompanied by orientation-dependent representations. This interpretation would explain why patients can recognize the objects (they are achieving orientation constancy by using the first of the two approaches described at the outset), but have lost access to the viewer-centered (or environment-centered) image representations that specify the object's orientation relative to them (or their environment). Turnbull and colleagues are pursuing this account while noting some difficulties with it: If object recognition is being achieved through orientation-invariant features or object-centered representations, then orientation agnosics should also be poor at discriminating the "handedness" of pictures—for example deciding whether two pictures are identical or are left-right reversed. Yet at least one orientation agnosic performed this task well (Turnbull, Beschin, & Della Salla, 1997). In addition, the orientation errors made by these patients are not random, but show a systematic preference for vertically aligned axes of elongation, with the flatter, more baselike end on the bottom (Turnbull, Beschin, & Della Salla, 1997). While not inconsistent with the operation of an isolated orientation-invariant system of shape representation, this error pattern is not explained by such a system either.

Finally, we do not yet know whether the preserved object representations in orientation agnosia are invariant over depth rotations. Would patients fail to discriminate the orientation of objects with different sides facing toward them? This would bear on the relevance of orientation agnosia to the spatial invariance of real-world object recognition. Davidoff

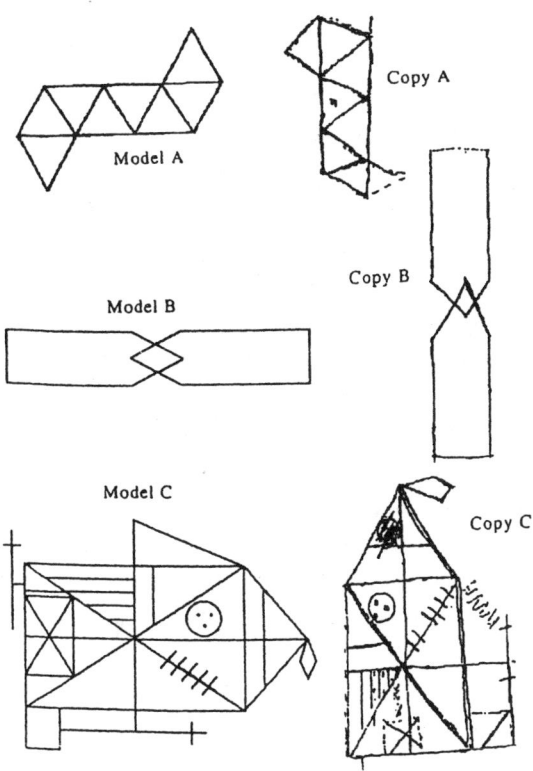

Figure 5.3
Geometric figures and copies of the figures made by an orientation agnosic studied by Turnbull, Laws, and McCarthy (1995).

and Warrington (1999) describe a patient who, like those of Turnbull and colleagues, is poor at judging picture orientation and handedness. He is also impaired in the recognition of the kinds of unusual views used to test perceptual categorization, as described in section 5.1. We might expect that preserved orientation-invariant representations, if invariant over changes in orientation along all axes, would permit such a patient to recognize depth-rotated objects. However as noted earlier, the unusual views test orientation invariance across particularly difficult spatial transformations or, when silhouetted, with reduced featural information. A more appropriate test for the present hypothesis would be the discrimination of real or artificial shapes rotated over a range of angular displacements. Further investigation of orientation agnosia will undoubtedly clarify these issues.

5.4   Orientation Constancy and Mental Rotation

The second of the two possible approaches to orientation constancy mentioned at the outset was mental rotation: one's current view of an object is mentally rotated to match a stored image. There is evidence that, at least in some circumstances, people use mental rotation when recognizing misoriented objects. Michael Tarr (Tarr & Pinker, 1989; Tarr, 1995) has pursued the issue with a systematic series of experiments in which normal subjects are taught to recognize novel objects presented at some, but not all, possible orientations during learning. For both two- and three-dimensional objects, subjects' response latencies to identifying the objects is a roughly linear function of the angular distance between the test item's orientation and nearest orientation seen during learning, consistent with a mental rotation process bringing the two representations into alignment. With drawings of real objects that have canonical orientations, subjects also show rotation–like response times as a function of the misorientation of the object, although the function flattens out with repeated exposure to the items (Jolicoeur, 1985). This suggests that both orientation-dependent and orientation-independent representations may play a role in normal object recognition (Jolicoeur, 1990). Recent imaging studies are consistent with this conclusion (Gauthier, Hayward, Tarr, Anderson, Skudlarski, & Gore, 2002; Vanrie, Beatse, Wagemans, Sunaert, & Van Hecke P, 2002), showing both common and distinctive patterns of activation for mental rotation and orientation normalization in object recognition.

One way to evaluate the role of mental rotation in orientation constancy is to investigate the effects of a loss of mental rotation ability on the recognition of misoriented objects. The study of such patients can address the question of whether mental rotation is a normal and essential part of object recognition.

Two case studies are directly relevant to this question, with converging support from a third. One patient, studied by Kate Hammond and myself, had severely impaired mental rotation ability following a large stroke that damaged much of his right parietal, frontal, and temporal lobes (Farah & Hammond, 1988). On three separate tests of mental rotation, he was able to perform the 0 degree control trials, but his performance was barely above chance when the stimuli were rotated as little as 45 degrees.

With real objects his visual recognition was unimpaired, and although his recognition of drawings was mildly impaired, he performed identically with inverted pictures (78 percent in both cases). He also was able to read upside down. He was even able to reinterpret letters according to their orientation—for example, looking at a Z and naming it as a Z in that orientation and also a sideways N. Another patient, described by Morton and Morris (1995), became poor at mental rotation following a left parieto-occipital stroke, yet retained good object recognition ability, including the ability to recognize unusual views.

The reverse dissociation has also been noted: Turnbull and McCarthy (1996) described a patient who had retained mental rotation ability despite impairment in the recognition of misoriented objects. Such a dissociation is inconsistent with the possibility that mental rotation tasks are simply harder tests of the same underlying ability as object constancy tasks, an alternative explanation of the previous two patients' performance. These cases suggest that mental rotation is not essential for object constancy; to the extent that it is used under normal circumstances, it is an ancillary or redundant process.

Chapter 6

Associative Visual Agnosia

Like the term "apperceptive agnosia," "associative agnosia" has been used quite broadly to cover a heterogeneous set of conditions. It includes impairments in general semantic knowledge and impairments confined to the naming (as opposed to the recognition) of visually presented objects, which are discussed in chapters 8 and 9. The more common and specific meaning of associative agnosia is a selective impairment in the recognition of visually presented objects, despite apparently adequate visual perception of them.

There are three criteria for membership in this category. The first is difficulty recognizing a variety of visually presented objects, as demonstrated by naming as well as such nonverbal tests of recognition such as grouping objects together according to their semantic category or gesturing to indicate their normal functions. The second criterion is normal recognition of objects through modalities other than vision—for example, by touching the object, hearing its characteristic sound, or being given a verbal definition of it. The third criterion is intact visual perception, or at least visual perception that seems adequate to the task of recognizing the object. This last criterion is usually tested by having patients copy objects or drawings that they cannot recognize.

6.1   Associative Visual Agnosia: A Case Description

A well-documented case of associative object agnosia was reported by Rubens and Benson in 1971. Their subject was a middle-aged man who had suffered an acute drop in blood pressure with resulting brain damage. His mental status and language abilities were normal, and his visual acuity was 20/30, with a right homonymous hemianopia (blindness in the right visual hemifield). His one severe impairment was an inability to recognize most visual stimuli.

For the first three weeks in the hospital the patient could not identify common objects presented visually and did not know what was on his plate until he tasted it. He identified objects immediately on touching them. When shown a stethoscope, he described it as "a long cord with a round thing at the end," and asked if it could be a watch. He identified a can opener as "could be a key." Asked to name a cigarette lighter, he said, "I don't know" but named it after the examiner lit it. He said he was "not sure" when shown a toothbrush. Asked to identify a comb, he said, "I don't know." When shown a large matchbook, he said, "It could be a container for keys." He correctly identifed glasses. For a pipe, he said, "Some type of utensil, I'm not sure." Shown a key, he said, "I don't know what that is; perhaps a file or a tool of some sort."

He was never able to describe or demonstrate the use of an object if he could not name it. If he misnamed an object his demonstration of its use would correspond to the mistaken identification. Identification improved very slightly when given the category of the object (e.g., "something to eat") or when asked to point to a named object instead of being required to give the name. When told the correct name of an object, he usually responded with a quick nod and said, "Yes, I see it now." Then, often he could point out various parts of the previously unrecognized item as readily as a normal subject (e.g., the stem and bowl of a pipe, and the laces, sole, and heel of a shoe). However, if asked by the examiner "Suppose I told you that the last object was not really a pipe, what would you say?" He would reply, "I would take your word for it. Perhaps it's not really a pipe." Similar vacillation never occurred with tactilely or aurally identified objects.

After three weeks on the ward, object naming ability had improved so that he could name many common objects, but this was variable; he might correctly name an object one time and misname it later. Performance deteriorated severely if any part of the object was covered by the examiner. He could match identical objects but not group objects by categories (clothing, food). He could draw the outlines of objects (key, spoon, etc.) which he could not identify. He was unable to recognize members of his family, the hospital staff, or even his own face in the mirror. . . . Sometimes he had difficulty distinguishing a line drawing of an animal's face from a man's face, but he always recognized it as a face.

Ability to recognize pictures of objects was greatly impaired, and after repeated testing he could name only one or two out of ten line drawings. He was always able to name geometrical forms (circle, square, triangle, cube). Remarkably, he could make excellent copies of line drawings and still fail to name the subject. . . . He easily matched drawings of objects that he could not identify, and had no difficulty discriminating between complex nonrepresentational patterns differing from each other only subtly. He occasionally failed in discriminating because he included imperfections in the paper or in the printer's ink. He could never group drawings by class unless he could first name the subject.

Reading, both aloud and for comprehension, was greatly limited. He could read, hesitantly, most printed letters, but often misread "K" as "R" and "L" as "T" and vice versa. . . . He was able to read words slowly by spelling them aloud. (Rubens & Benson, 1971, pp. 308–309).

6.2   General Characteristics of Associative Visual Agnosia

Although associative visual agnosia is a relatively rare disorder, it is also relatively likely to be written up when observed, and the literature therefore contains many detailed case reports. Representative cases that show the same overall pattern of spared and impaired visual abilities as Rubens and Benson's case include Albert, Reches, and Silverberg (1975); Bauer (1982); Butter and Trobe, 1994; Davidoff and Wilson (1985; also Wilson & Davidoff, 1993); DeRenzi and Lucchelli (1993); Hecaen and Ajuriaguerra (1956); Levine (1978); Levine and Calvanio (1989); Moscovitch, Winocur, and Behrmann (1997), R. A. McCarthy and Warrington (1986), Pillon, Signoret, and Lhermitte (1981); Ratcliff and Newcombe (1982); Riddoch and Humphreys (1987a); and Wapner, Judd, and Gardner (1978). These patients cannot reliably name visually presented objects, and when they hazard an incorrect guess, it is often a visually similar object, as when the patient described above called a can opener "a key" and a key as "a file or a tool of some sort." Recognition is no better when tested nonverbally, for example in a sorting task where related objects must be grouped together (e.g., a baseball mitt, and a baseball, a paring knife and an apple). Yet in some ways the perceptual abilities of these patients are impressively good.

Tests of visual spatial processing are generally performed successfully. Indeed, it was the preservation of visual spatial processing in associative visual agnosics, contrasted with the preservation of visual object recognition but poor spatial processing in dorsal simultanagnosics, that first suggested the existence of separate "what" and "where" visual processing streams (see Ungerleider & Mishkin, 1982). For example, Rubens and Benson's

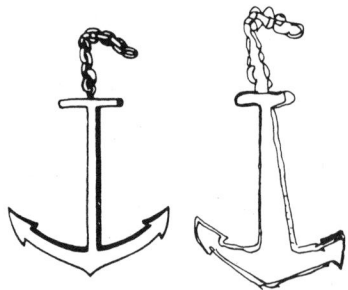

Figure 6.1
Drawing of an anchor that an associative agnosic could not recognize, and his copy (from Ratcliff & Newcombe, 1982).

(1971) patient performed well on a number of clinical tests of spatial ability including a visual maze. I have tested the agnosic patient LH on a number of challenging tests of spatial ability, including the mental rotation of three-dimensional shapes and the recall of spatial relations among American states, and can report that he does substantially better than me.

The visual-spatial prowess of agnosic patients is not that surprising given that the tasks in question make minimal demands on the ability to represent object appearance. More surprising is their copying ability. Figures 6.1 and 6.2 show the impressive copies made by two associative agnosic patients of drawings they could not recognize. This would seem to imply that their perception of these drawings is normal, or at least sufficient to allow recognition. Whether this is in fact true has implications for the nature of the conputations underlying visual object recognition, as discussed next.

6.3   A Perceptual or a Mnemonic Impairment?

Visual recognition requires that memory be searched for a representation that resembles the current stimulus input. The way that recognition occurs in a conventional, or Von Neumann, computer is that a representation of the input is compared to representations stored in memory, using an explicit comparison process that is itself part of a stored program in the computer. The process is analogous to taking the title or call number of a book that you have written on a piece of paper, and searching the library

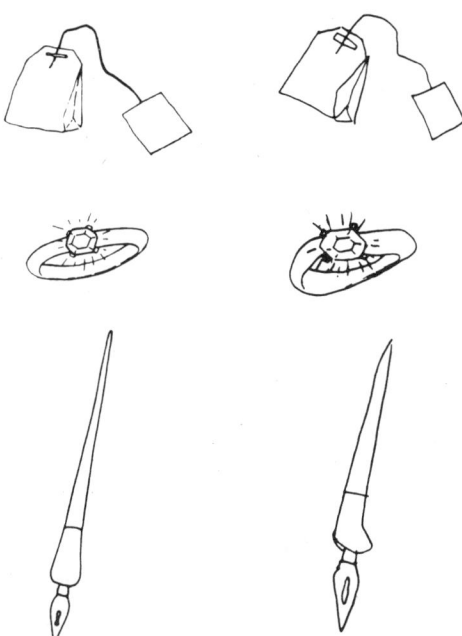

Figure 6.2
Three drawings that an associative agnosic could not recognize, and his copies of those drawings (from Farah et al., 1988).

shelves to find the same title or call number written on the spine of the book. In terms of visual object recognition, perceptual processes would culminate in a high-level perceptual representation of the stimulus, which would then be compared with stored memory representations of stimuli. When a match is found, the associated semantic knowledge of the object is then available, just as the contents of the book become available once the title has been located on the shelf. An important feature of the computer, library, and object recognition scenarios is the existence of two tokens of the item being recognized, one that has been derived from the input and one that resides in memory.

On the assumption that human visual object recognition has this much in common with Von Neumann computers, a natural question to ask is: Does agnosia result from a loss of high-level perceptual representations, or of stored memory representations? The visual perceptual abilities of associative agnosic patients seem relevant to answering this question, in that an agnosic patient who could pass all visual perceptual tests with flying colors would presumably have lost the stored visual memory representations of objects. However, despite the many impressively copied drawings to be found in the literature, including those in figures 6.1 and 6.2, close scrutiny invariably reveals significant perceptual abnormalities in agnosic patients.

For example, although the final products of patients' copying may look very good, the manner in which they are produced is strikingly abnormal. "Slavish," "line-by-line," and "piecemeal" are often used in describing the manner of copying in these cases (e.g., Moscovitch, Winocur, & Behrmann, 1997; Butter & Trobe, 1994; Ratcliff & Newcombe, 1982; Wapner, Judd, & Gardner, 1978; Brown, 1972). I watched as a patient drew the pen, tea bag, and ring shown in figure 6.2, and can report that they were indeed executed very slowly, with many pauses to check the correspondence of each line of the copy and the original. Of course, one must allow for the fact that the patient did not recognize the objects, and was therefore in effect drawing a nonsense figure. Nevertheless, his technique seemed abnormally slow and piecemeal. Although the patient of DeRenzi and Luccelli (1993) did not strike the authors as being especially slow in her copying, her performance on an overlapping figures task was poor, and also particularly informative on the role of object recognition in the performance of "perceptual" tasks. When meaningless shapes were substituted for object drawings in the overlapping figures task, the gap between normal and patient performance did not diminish, implying that her ability to see familiar objects was indeed impaired.

Other observations of agnosic patients are also consistent with an impairment in visual perception. Such patients are abnormally sensitive to the visual quality of stimuli, performing best with real objects, next best with photographs, and worst with line drawings, an ordering reflecting increasing impoverishment of the stimulus. Tachistoscopic presentation, which also reduces visual stimulus quality, also impairs associative agnosics' performance dramatically. As already mentioned, the vast majority of their recognition errors are visual in nature, that is, they correspond to an object of similar shape rather than a semantically related object or an object with a similar-sounding name. For example, on four different occasions when I asked an associative agnosic to name a picture of a baseball bat, he made four different errors, each reflecting shape similarity: paddle, knife, baster, thermometer. In some cases errors that are classified as semantic might equally well have been classified as visual—for example "Pegasus" for centaur and "Taj Mahal" for pagoda (Wilson & Davidoff, 1993). If the underlying impairment were in the visual processing of the stimulus, it seems intuitively plausible that the resulting errors would be "near misses" in visual similarity space. Although in a sufficiently interactive system, visual errors can be accounted for by impaired access to semantic knowledge (Hinton & Shallice, 1991), such accounts predict accompanying semantic errors. Therefore, for those cases in which visual shape errors are found in the absence of semantic errors, it is likely that visual shape perception is at fault.

One conclusion that could be drawn on the basis of these observations is that perception is at fault in all cases of associative agnosia so far studied. However, there is an alternative way to view the evidence on perception in associative agnosia, according to which the question "Perception or memory?" is simply the wrong question.

Recall that the distinction between the stimulus-derived and the stored representations is a required aspect of recognition in information-processing systems based on Von Neumann computation. However, there are other ways of implementing information processing in which recognition does not involve two distinct tokens of the item to be recognized. These are found in neural network-based systems.

In neural networks, representations correspond to activation of certain neuronlike units, which are interconnected in a network. The extent to which the activation of one unit causes an increase or decrease in the activation of a neighboring unit depends on the "weight" of the connection between them; positive weights cause units to excite each other, and negative weights cause units to inhibit each other. Upon presentation of the input pattern to the input units, all of the units connected with those input units will begin to change their activation under the influence of two kinds of constraints: the activation value of the units to which they are connected and the weights on the connections. These units might in turn connect to others, and influence their activation levels in the same way. In recurrent, or attractor, networks the units downstream will also begin to influence the activation levels of the earlier units. Eventually, these shifting activation levels across the units of the network settle into a stable pattern of activation, which is the representation that corresponds to the recognized object. That pattern is determined jointly by the input activation (the stimulus input) and the weights of the network (the system's knowledge of all objects).

The two ways of implementing recognition are so different that it is difficult to compare them except at a very abstract level. For instance, one can say that the system's knowledge in a conventional computer's implementation of recognition consists of separate stored representations of the stimulus and the comparison procedure, whereas in a neural network it consists just of the connection weights, which store knowledge of object appearance and carry out the search process. In both types of system there is a distinction between the early representations of the stimulus, closer to the input level, and the high-level object representations that underlie object recognition. But there are two tokens of the high-level representation involved in conventional systems, the "perceptual" representation derived from the stimulus and the stored "memory" representation, whereas there is only one token in neural networks. Distinctions such as "structure versus process" and "perception versus memory," which seem almost logically necessary when one is thinking in terms of Von Neumann computation, dissolve when one considers the neural network implementation of memory search.

6.4 Object Representation in Associative Visual Agnosia

Whether the highest levels of object representation involve distinct perceptual and mnemonic tokens or a single perceptual-mnemonic representation, we can ask what kinds of information are encoded in them. By characterizing the nature of the missing information in associative agnosics' representations, we will learn about the kinds of visual information that must be extracted from the object image to enable recognition.

Surprisingly little systematic research has addressed this question. Furthermore, what little there is must be interpreted with the awareness that not all results necessarily apply to all patients. It is possible that visual representation can be impaired in several different ways and lead to the same general constellation of abilities and deficits characteristic of associative visual agnosia. In the next section, I will argue that this is indeed the case.

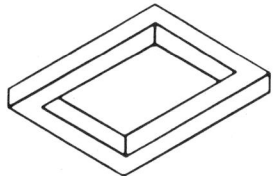

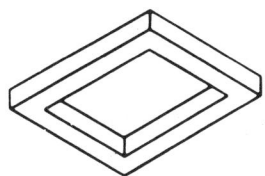

Figure 6.3
Possible and impossible figures of the kind used in Ratcliff and Newcombe's (1982) study of object vision in associative visual agnosia.

Investigations of visual representation in associative agnosia have generally involved patients whose agnosia extends to faces, and have revealed disproportionate problems with the global structure of complex objects, relative to simpler shapes or simpler parts of shapes. Ratcliff and Newcombe (1982) conducted an early investigation of perceptual processing in associative agnosia and, using possible and impossible shapes of the kind shown in figure 6.3, found a loss of global or "gestalt" perception. Although both possible and impossible shapes are normal at the level of local parts, the parts of an impossible shape cannot be assigned a three-dimensional interpretation that is consistent throughout the shape. Discriminating between possible and impossible shapes therefore requires seeing the overall structure of the shape. Ratcliff and Newcombe found that an associative visual agnosic who was able to copy the two kinds of shapes was nevertheless unable to distinguish between them. The patient of DeRenzi and Lucchelli (1993) was similarly unable to distinguish possible and impossible figures despite good perceptual function by some criteria.

Levine and Calvanio (1989) analyzed the perception of an associative visual agnosic patient using the factor-analyzed test kit of Ekstrom, French, and Harman (1976). They found that most of the perceptual factors measured in the test battery were reasonably preserved in their patient. The patient's most severe impairments were found on those tests which measure "visual closure," the ability to perceive the shape and identity of an object that has been fragmented or degraded by visual noise. When local shape information is missing or distorted, recognition depends on the extraction of the overall form, as in the pictures shown in figure 6.4.

The concept of "integrative agnosia," proposed by Riddoch and Humphreys (1987a), is based on a more explicit and specific claim about the nature of the object representation impairment. They, too, observed the difficulty of at least some agnosic patients with more global shape representation, and suggested a specific interpretation for this difficulty in terms of the impaired integration of local shape parts into higher-order shapes. This hypothesis was suggested by the observation that when agnosic patients guess the identity of objects or pictures they cannot recognize, they often base their guess on a single local feature. For example, an animal with a long, tapered tail might engender "rat" or "mouse" as a guess. A baby carriage, with metal spokes inside the wheels, might be called a "bicycle." This behavior invites interpretation in terms of a hierarchical system of shape representation, whose lower-level part representations are relatively intact but whose higher-level integration of the parts is damaged or unavailable. Riddoch and Humphreys (1987a) introduced the term "integrative agnosia" for such cases.

In addition to the use of local parts for guessing the identity of objects, Riddoch and Humphreys collected additional evidence from their patient, HJA, that seemed consistent with this interpretation: impaired recognition of briefly presented stimuli (because, they argue, if parts are serially encoded, more time will be required); impaired recognition of overlapping drawings (because impaired part integration will be further taxed by the possibility of misconjoining the parts of different objects); impaired discrimination of real objects from pseudo objects composed of mismatched parts of real objects; and greater impairment (relative to normal subjects) in recognizing more complex depictions (because these contain more parts). Butter and Trobe (1994) replicated many of these observations with another associative visual agnosic.

It is true that an impairment in integrating local shape parts into global wholes is consistent with the findings just listed. However, such an impairment is not the only way to account for these findings. First con-

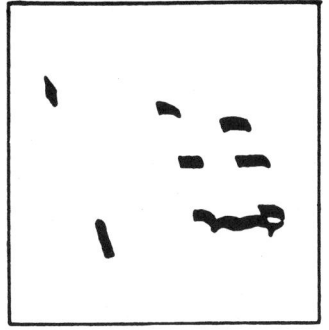 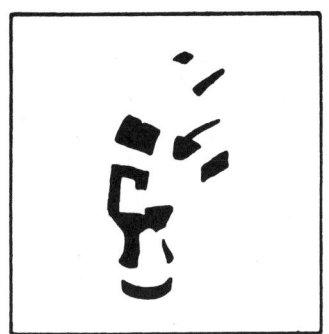

rⁿ̃₁c̃n̄tₒ

c̄ᵍₛ\

ⁿ̃ː̃ε̃ⁿ̃ₗ̃

Figure 6.4
Items testing visual closure from the Ekstrom et al. (1976) battery of factor-referenced tests.

sider the basic finding that agnosics may guess the identity of objects based on a single correctly perceived part. While consistent with an impairment in integration of parts, it is also consistent with almost any type impairment in shape-processing capacity, since the shape of a part will always be simpler than the shape of a whole object. Above and beyond this, in any system for which there is a fixed probability of recognizing a given shape (part or whole), there will be more successes with just parts than with just wholes, simply because parts are more numerous.

The other features of integrative agnosia are similarly ambiguous with respect to the underlying impairment in shape representation. The slower speed of agnosic object recognition is hardly a unique prediction of impaired part integration. Nor is the detrimental effect of overlapping pictures, since almost any impairment of shape representation one can think of would make it less robust to interfering contours. Similarly, object decision would be expected to be impaired whenever shape perception is defective in any way. The difference in performance between silhouettes and detailed drawings after unspecified perceptual impairment could take the form of better performance the more information is available (hence drawings better than silhouettes) or better performance the simpler the shape to be perceived (hence silhouttes better than drawings), but certainly the latter prediction is not unique to a specific impairment of part integration.

The ambiguity of these data is at least in part due to the fact that with real objects or their depictions, one cannot cleanly manipulate one type of visual information without affecting other types. For example, silhouetting a shape, or deleting or changing its features, also changes the gestalt. Breaking the gestalt by scrambling features introduces new, emergent features at the picture's "seams."

Perhaps motivated by this problem, Rentschler, Treutwein, and Landis (1994) took a different approach to assessing local and global form perception. They operationalized global or gestalt perception by testing the perception of textures and moire patterns, and operationalized local or featural perception by testing the perception of individual texture elements. Impaired perception was found in both of the patients they tested, but the nature of the impairment differed. The patient with face recognition difficulty could discriminate between texture elements such as those shown in figure 6.5a, but not between texture displays such as those in figure 6.5b. She was also impaired at the discrimination of strong and weak moire patterns such as those shown in figure 6.6. The other patient, who was able to recognize faces, was poor at discriminating texture elements, and therefore also their global organization (figure 6.5a and b), but performed normally with moire patterns, whose local elements are dots and whose discrimination therefore depends solely on global shape (figure 6.6). Had they merely assessed the perception of global structure with the stimulus whose local elements have shape, shown in figure 6.5b, the investigators would have reached conclusions very similar to those of previous authors: a single problem with the extraction of global structure.

a

b

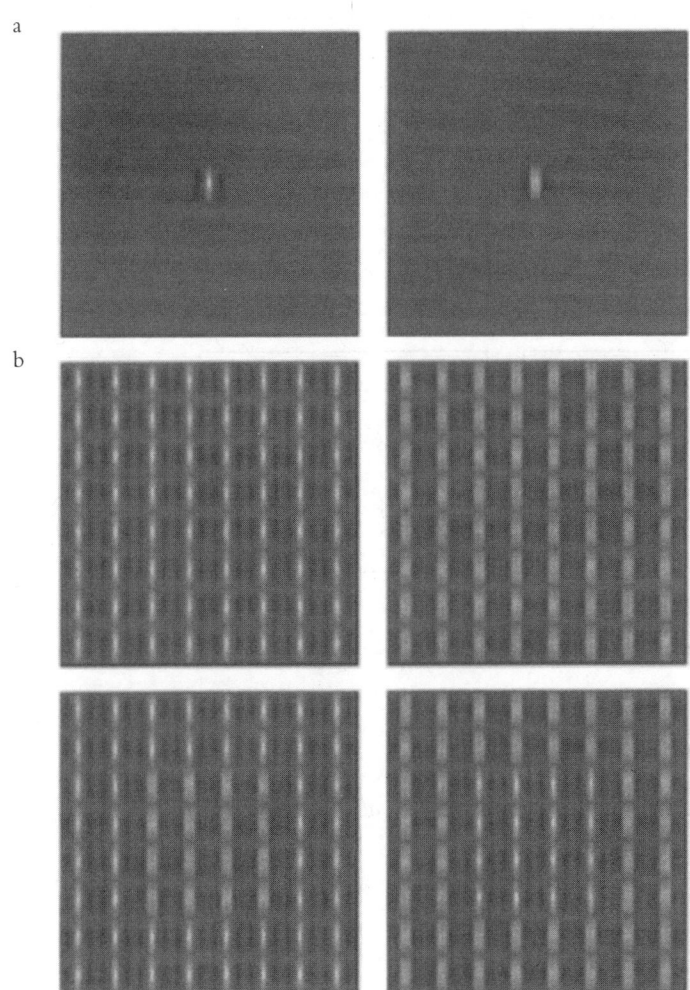

Figure 6.5
Texture displays used in Rentschler, Treutwein, and Landis' (1994) study of visual perception in associative agnosia.

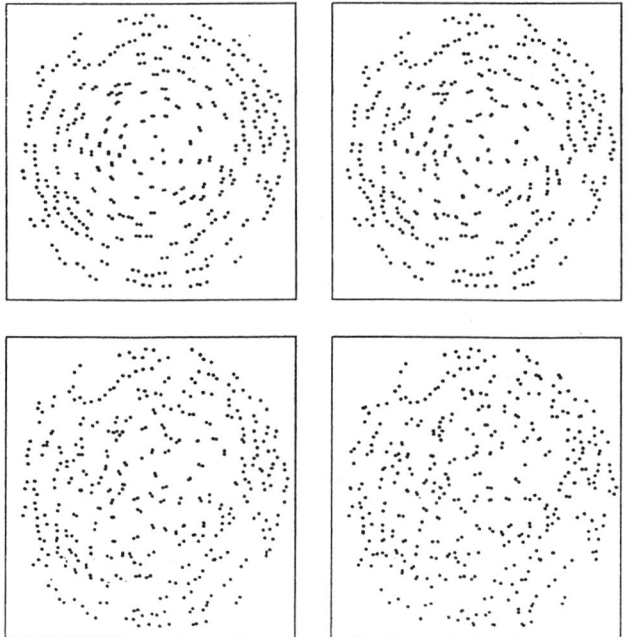

Figure 6.6
Moire patterns used in a study of visual perception in associative agnosia.

6.5   Delineating the Subsystems of Visual Recognition

The scope of the recognition impairment in associative visual agnosia is variable, sometimes affecting all visual stimuli, sometimes affecting just faces, and sometimes sparing faces or printed words. This suggests that more than one underlying recognition system can be impaired in associative visual agnosia, and raises the question: How many different systems are there for visual recognition, and how do they differ in their representation of visual stimuli?

The pairwise dissociability of both face and written word recognition from object recognition more generally might seem to imply that there are three corresponding types of visual recognition ability. However, this three-part organization for visual recognition would follow only if all possible *triads* of spared and impaired recognition of faces, objects, and words were observed. When I tabulated the face, word, and object recognition of ninety-nine associative visual agnosics whose case reports were

indexed on Medline between 1966 and 1988, I found that certain combinations of these abilities were not observed (Farah, 1991). Specifically,
there were no well-documented cases in which the recognition of common objects was impaired while the recognition of both faces and words
was spared, and a similar lack of cases in which the recognition of both
faces and words was impaired but the recognition of objects was spared.

This pattern is of interest because it suggests that there are just two,
rather than three, underlying systems of visual representation: one system
that is necessary for printed word recognition, used for object recognition,
and not used for face recognition, and another system that is necessary for
face recognition, used for object recognition, and not used for printed
word recognition.

Any broad and sweeping generalization in science is an invitation,
to oneself and to others, to search for disconfirming instances. Three such
instances have been put forward to challenge the "two systems" view. My
colleagues Buxbaum, Glosser, and Coslett (1999) studied a patient whose
prosopagnosia and pure alexia ought to have been accompanied by object
agnosia, according to the hypothesis. The patient was able to recognize the
real, three-dimensional objects in his environment, which admittedly
rules out a severe object agnosia. However, I think the title of their report, "Impaired Face and Word Recognition Without Object Agnosia,"
overstates the case, since the patient was able to name only 78 percent of
drawings with 60 seconds viewing time for each, and his errors were all
visual in nature.

A different type of disconfirmation is offered by patients with an isolated object recognition impairment, in the absence of prosopagnosia or
alexia. Two cases of relevance to this prediction have been reported. In
the first, Rumiati, Humphreys, Riddoch, and Bateman (1994) described a
patient who, in the course of a dementing illness, was described as neither
prosopagnosic nor alexic but performed poorly on a number of tests of object processing. However, many aspects of the case were unclear, including whether his object recognition was impaired at all! His difficulties with
object knowledge also were present with purely verbal tasks, further un-
dermining the relevance of this case to the hypothesis in question. The authors and I subsequently discussed these issues in print (Farah, 1997a,
1997b; Rumiati & Humphreys, 1997). In a more recent report this group
presents another case of, in the words of their title, "Agnosia Without

Prosopagnosia or Alexia," yet again I question its relevance, given that the patient consistently performed below normal limits when her knowledge about objects was tested through reading (Humphreys & Rumiati, 1998). In both cases the patient's impairments seem to include semantic levels of representation, which limits their usefulness in testing theories of vision.

6.6   Characterizing the Subsystems of Visual Recognition

How do the hypothesized two visual recognition systems differ, aside from their involvement in face and word recognition? Evidence is accumulating that the systems differ in the way shape is represented. In one system, a complex shape is broken into parts, with the result that a larger number of relatively simpler parts must be represented. In the other system, there is little or no part decomposition, with the result that a small number of relatively complex parts must be represented. Much of the relevant evidence comes from research on the recognition of faces, objects, and printed words in normal subjects. This evidence will be summarized briefly here.

One way of measuring the relative contribution of part and whole information in face recognition is based on the finding that, when a portion of a pattern corresponds to a part in the natural parse of the pattern by the visual system, it will be better remembered. Recognition of an isolated portion thus provides an assay for the degree to which a portion of a pattern is treated as a psychologically real part by the viewer. Tanaka and Farah (1993) taught subjects to identify faces and various contrasting classes of nonface stimuli, and then assessed the degree to which the parts of these stimuli were explicitly represented in subjects' memories. For example, in one experiment illustrated in figure 6.7, subjects learned to name a set of faces (e.g., Joe, Larry, etc.), as well as a set of houses (Bill's house, Tom's house, etc.). Subjects were then given two-alternative forced-choice tests of the identity of isolated parts (e.g., "Which is Joe's nose?" "Which is Bill's door?") or whole patterns in which the correct and incorrect choices differ only by a single part (e.g., "Which is Joe?" when confronted with Joe and a version of Joe with the alternative nose from the isolated-part test pair; "Which is Bill's house?" when confronted with Bill's house and a version of Bill's house with the alternative door from the isolated test pair). We found that, relative to their ability to recognize the

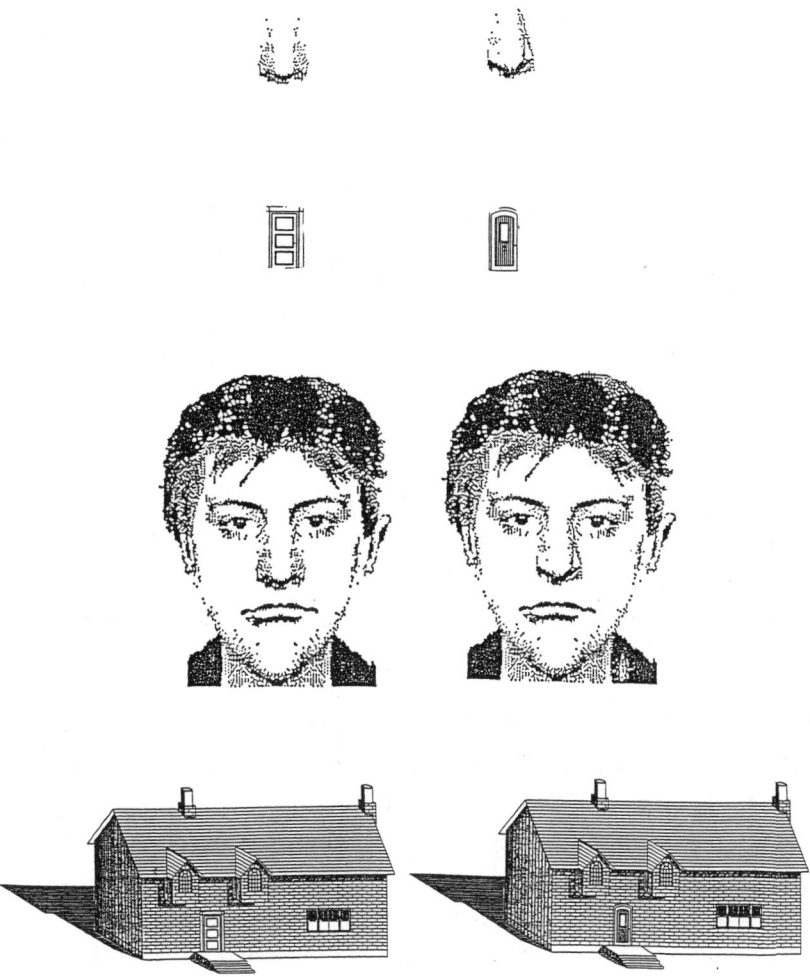

Figure 6.7
Examples of training and test stimuli from Tanaka and Farah's (1993) study of face perception.

whole faces and houses, subjects were impaired at recognizing parts of faces compared to parts of houses. Could the difference be caused by the nature of the parts themselves? No, because the same pattern of results was obtained when faces were compared to scrambled faces and inverted faces, whose parts are identical.

Tanaka and Sengco (1997) showed that these results should not be interpreted simply in terms of a part-based representation in which, for faces, the configuration of parts is particularly important. If this were the case, changes in configuration would affect overall face recognition, but so long as individual parts are explicitly represented, this manipulation should not affect the recognition of the individual parts per se. Testing this prediction by comparing upright faces to inverted faces and houses, they again found evidence of holistic coding of upright faces. The results of these experiments are consistent by the following hypothesis: during the learning and subsequent recognition of the houses, scrambled faces, and inverted faces, subjects explicitly represented their parts, whereas during the learning and subsequent recognition of the intact upright faces they did not, or they did so to a lesser extent.

Another way in which we have tested the holistic representation hypothesis is by seeing whether it could explain the face inversion effect (Farah, Tanaka, & Drain, 1995). If face recognition differs from other forms of object recognition by the use of relatively undecomposed or holistic representations, then perhaps the face inversion effect results from the use of holistic, or nonpart-based, representation. In the first experiment we taught subjects to identify random dot patterns and later tested their recognition of the patterns either upright or inverted. Half of the patterns learned by subjects were presented in a way that encouraged parsing the pattern into parts: each portion of the pattern corresponding to a part was a distinctive color, so that grouping by color defined parts. The other half of the patterns learned were presented in all black, and the test stimuli for all patterns were presented in black. When subjects had been induced to see the patterns in terms of parts during learning, their later performance at identifying the patterns showed no effect of orientation. In contrast, when they were not induced to encode the patterns in terms of parts, they showed an inversion effect in later recognition.

In a second experiment on the inversion effect, we manipulated subjects' encoding of faces and then tested their ability to recognize the faces upright and inverted. Subjects were induced to learn half of the faces in a partwise manner, by presenting them in the "exploded" format described earlier, whereas the other half of the faces to be learned were presented in a normal format. All faces were tested in a normal format. For the faces that were initially encoded in terms of parts, there was no inversion effect. In contrast, faces encoded normally showed a normal inversion effect. These results suggest that what is special about face recognition, by virtue of which it is so sensitive to orientation, is that it involves representations with relatively little or no part decomposition.

In another series of experiments we assessed the degree of part decomposition on-line during the perception of faces, using two types of experimental paradigm (Farah, Wilson, Drain, & Tanaka, 1998). In the first, we measured the relative availability of part and whole representations by requiring subjects to compare single features of simultaneously presented pairs of faces, and observed the influence of irrelevant features on their ability to judge the similarity or difference of the probed feature. For example, they might be asked whether two faces have the same or different noses. To the extent that subjects have explicit representations of the separate features of a face, then they should be able to compare them with one another. To the extent that they do not have explicit representations of these features, but only a holistic representation of the entire face, they should experience cross talk from irrelevant features when judging the probed feature. The amount of cross talk with upright faces was significantly more than with inverted faces, suggesting that the relative availability of parts and wholes differed for the two orientations, with parts less available in upright faces.

In three additional experiments we explored the effect on face perception of masks composed of face parts or whole faces. As Johnston and McClelland (1980) reasoned in their experiments on word perception, to the extent that masks contain shape elements similar to those used in representing the stimulus, the mask will interfere with perception of the stimulus. The effects of part and whole masks on the perception of upright faces were compared to their effects on the perception of words, inverted faces, and houses. In all cases, part masks were relatively less disruptive than whole masks for upright face perception, when compared to the effects of part and whole masks on the perception of words, inverted faces, and houses.

To return to the "two systems" view of agnosia, the foregoing results from normal subjects suggest the following: If the representation of parts is only mildly impaired, then most objects will be recognized, and only those objects which undergo little or no decomposition into parts, and whose parts are therefore relatively complex, will be affected. This corresponds to prosopagnosia. If the representation of parts is more severely impaired, then the recognition deficit will extend to more objects, and only objects with the simplest parts will be recognized. This corresponds to object agnosia with prosopagnosia but without alexia. If the ability to represent parts is intact, but the ability to rapidly encode multiple parts is impaired, then most objects will be recognized. The only objects that will be affected will be those which undergo decomposition into many parts, and for which multiple parts must be encoded before recognition can occur. This corresponds to alexia. If the impairment in this ability is severe enough that even a moderate number of parts cannot be rapidly and accurately encoded, then the recognition of objects other than words will be affected as well. However, even in this case faces should not be affected, since they do not require encoding multiple separate parts. This corresponds to agnosia with alexia but without prosopagnosia. If both abilities are impaired, then the recognition of all objects will be affected. This corresponds to agnosia with both alexia and prosopagnosia.

6.7 Neuropathology of Associative Visual Agnosia

Associative visual agnosia is most frequently seen after bilateral infarction of the posterior cerebral arteries, but is occasionally the result of other etiologies, such as head injury, and is also sometimes seen with unilateral lesions. If one considers all cases meeting the criteria for associative visual agnosia together, it is difficult to identify a critical lesion site. Most cases have bilateral occipitotemporal lesions, but many well-documented cases have either left or right unilateral lesions.

The variability in lesion sites might signify the existence of more than one underlying type of associative agnosia, and indeed the neuropathology becomes more systematic when one subdivides the cases according to the "two systems" view described in section 6.5. When the cases are arranged in terms of their presumed impairments in parts-based and holistic object representation, a clear pattern emerges.

A selective impairment in parts-based representation is the result of unilateral left temporo-occipital damage. Depending on severity, patients are either pure alexics or alexic and object agnosic, but invariably show intact face recognition, since face recognition is not dependent on parts-based recognition. Both pure alexia and agnosia sparing faces are associated with unilateral left temporo-occipital damage (Feinberg et al., 1994). A selective impairment in holistic representation can be the result of unilateral right, or bilateral, temporo-occipital damage. Depending on severity, patients are either prosopagnosic or prosopagnosic and object agnosic, but invariably can read, since word recognition is not dependent on holistic representation. Although most cases of prosopagnosia involve bilateral lesions, a considerable number involve unilateral lesions of the right hemisphere, consistent with a right hemisphere dominance for this ability that varies among individuals from relative to absolute. In less strongly lateralized individuals, the remaining left hemisphere capability would enable recognition after a right hemisphere lesion, and therefore only bilateral lesions will result in a noticeable impairment, whereas in more strongly lateralized individuals a unilateral right hemisphere lesion will suffice (DeRenzi, Perani, Carlesimo, Silveri, & Fazio, 1994). Impairment in both parts-based and holistic shape representation would therefore be expected only after bilateral lesions, and would be manifest as an across-the-board agnosia for faces, objects, and printed words. In such cases, the lesions are indeed bilateral (Farah, 1991).

Chapter 7

Prosopagnosia and Topographic Agnosia

7.1 Modules and "Special" Systems

As cognitive science emerged from the fields of psychology, computer science, and linguistics in the 1970s, it defined its main scientific business as characterizing the "functional architecture" of cognition (e.g., Pylyshyn, 1981). "Architecture" conveyed its emphasis on the large-scale structure of the cognitive system and was suggestive of a structure with clearly demarcated components. A general issue that arose in this context was how extensively parcelated the structure was. On one side of the issue were advocates of "unified architectures," which accomplished a wide range of cognitive functions using a relatively small number of general-purpose cognitive components (e.g., Anderson, 1983; Newell, 1990; McClelland & Rumelhart, 1981). On the other side were advocates of "modular architectures," which consisted of many special-purpose components that carry out specific functions (Barkow, Cosmides, & Tooby, 1992; Fodor, 1982; Gardner, 1983). While the unified architectures had parsimony in their favor, the modular architectures found support in linguistics and biology.

Chomsky and his followers argued that language was "special," by which they meant that language learning and language use did not depend on the same mental systems used for other types of learning, perception, and cognition. Fodor's (1983) book, *The Modularity of Mind,* drew its examples mainly from psycholinguistics. Evolutionary biopsychologists argued that natural selection would most likely create a modular mind, because specific solutions to specific problems in our evolutionary past were more likely to occur by chance than were general-purpose solutions.

Neuropsychologists documented highly selective impairments in cognition that were most easily explained as the loss of a specialized module.

Among the selective impairments in visual neuropsychology are face recognition and topographic disorientation. Face recognition, in particular, has been a focus of the modularity debate.

7.2   Prosopagnosia: A Case Description

Prosopagnosia is the inability to recognize faces despite intact intellectual functioning and even apparently intact visual recognition of most other stimuli. Bodamer introduced the term "prosopagnosia" in 1947, in conjunction with a careful study of three cases, and many cases have been reported in the neurological literature since then. A particularly complete description of a prosopagnosic patient is given by Pallis (1955):

He was of above average intelligence and his general level of awareness was extremely keen. His memory was remarkable. . . . His span of digit retention was 8 forward and 6 backwards. There was no hesitation in his speech and he could obey complex orders. He read smoothly and there was no trouble in understanding and later describing what he had read. . . . He promptly recognized, named, and demonstrated the use of a wide variety of test objects. . . . The significance of line drawings was immediately apparent to him, and he could accurately describe the content of various pictures he was shown.

He mixed readily with the other patients on the ward, but rarely spoke unless spoken to first. He could not identify his medical attendants. "You must be a doctor because of your white coat, but I don't know which one you are. I'll know if you speak." He failed to identify his wife during visiting hours. She was told one day, without his possible knowledge, to walk right past his bed, but he did not show the least sign of recognition. Repeated attempts were made to "catch him out" but none succeeded. If the disability was a feigned one, it was a performance of quite unbelievable virtuosity and consistency. . . . He failed to identify pictures of Mr. Churchill, Mr. Aneurin Bevan, Hitler, Stalin, Miss Marilyn Monroe, or Mr. Groucho Marx. When confronted with such portraits he would proceed deductively, analyzing one feature after another, searching for the "critical detail" which would yield the answer. In human faces, this was rarely forthcoming. There was somewhat less difficulty with animal faces. A goat was eventually recognized by its ears and beard, a giraffe by its neck, a crocodile by its dentition, and a cat by its whiskers. . . .

The patient had analysed his difficulty in identifying faces with considerable insight. "I can see the eyes, nose, and mouth quite clearly, but they just don't add up. They all seem chalked in, like on a blackboard. . . . I have to tell by the clothes or by the voice whether it is a man or a woman. . . . The hair may help a lot, or if there is a mustache. . . .

"At the club I saw someone strange staring at me, and asked the steward who it was. You'll laugh at me. I'd been looking at myself in a mirror."

7.3   General Characteristics of Prosopagnosia

Many other cases of prosopagnosia have been reported in the literature, including Assal, Favre, and Anderes (1984); Bornstein and Kidron (1959); Cole and Perez-Cruet (1964); De Renzi (1986); De Renzi, Faglioni, Grossi, and Nichelli (1991); Farah, Levinson, and Klein (1995); M. C. Kay and Levin (1982); Lhermitte and Pillon (1975); McNeil and Warrington (1993); Nardelli, Buonanno, Coccia, Fiaschi, Terzian, and Rizzuto (1982); Sergent and Signoret (1992); Shuttleworth, Syring, and Allen (1982); Takahashi, Kawamura, Hirayama, Shiota, and Isono (1995), and Whitely and Warrington (1977). Particularly in the more recent reports, different patients are contrasted with one another, and correspondingly different forms of prosopagnosia are proposed (De Renzi et al., 1991; McNeil & Warrington, 1991; Sergent & Signoret, 1992). Although there are unquestionably differences among the patients we label "prosopagnosic," and some of these differences may have important implications for conclusions we draw from the study of such patients, there are also many generalities. Therefore, at the risk of blurring some potentially important differences, I will focus on the generalities in the present discussion.

Agnosia for faces can be strikingly complete. Patients with associative visual agnosia for objects are typically able to recognize at least some objects under natural conditions in their environment, and show truly chance performance only when recognition is made more difficult by limiting viewing time, choosing uncommon objects, or presenting line drawings instead of real objects. In contrast, prosopagnosics may fail to recognize a single face reliably. Even their closest friends and family members may not be recognized until they speak. The utter lack of face recognition is apparent in the experience of Pallis's patient at his club, and in a very similar story related to me by a prosopagnosic acquaintance. This highly

educated and intelligent man was attending a conference held at a busy ho-
tel. Coming back from the men's room, he rounded a corner and found
himself walking toward someone. He found the man's behavior bizarre.
The man was staring at him and heading directly toward him. A few seconds later he realized he was facing a mirror.

As with Pallis's patient, most prosopagnosics complain of an alteration in the appearance of faces. Although they have no difficulty perceiving that a face is a face (and do not generally mistake wives for hats),
they often speak of seeing the parts individually and losing the whole or
gestalt. In a survey of published cases, Shuttleworth, Syring, and Allen
(1982) noted that in 85 percent of forty-four cases, patients had subjective visual complaints. A common objective test of face perception developed by Benton and Van Allen (1968) is the Test of Facial Recognition.
This task consists of a series of photographs of unfamiliar faces, viewed
from the front, each of which must be matched with one of a set of six
other photographs. Some of these sets of six photographs have been taken
from a different angle or under different lighting conditions. Examples
are shown in figure 7.1.

How do prosopagnosics perform on this stringent test of face perception? There is a range of performance across different cases, and different authors focus on different portions of this range. For example, Damasio
(1985) cites the research of Benton and Van Allen (e.g., 1972; Benton,
1980) in support of the claim that these patients' "perception of both the
whole and the parts of a facial stimulus is intact. . . . Prosopagnosic patients
are generally able to perform complex perceptual tasks (such as the Benton and Van Allen test of unfamiliar facial discrimination)" (p. 263).
Benton and Van Allen's (1972) statement is somewhat less strong: "The
disabilities underlying prosopagnosia and impairment in performance on
the visuoperceptive task of discriminating unfamiliar faces are, or at least
may be, dissociable" (p. 170). This conclusion was based on a review of
three cases of prosopagnosia, one of which was "markedly impaired" at
discriminating faces and two of which were "essentially normal" (p. 168),
as well a new case, who performed "on a mediocre level, but within broad
normal limits" (p. 169) on their test of face discrimination.

The interpretation of patients' performance on this task must be further qualified by a consideration of the speed and manner of task completion. Newcombe (1979) observed a prosopagnosic patient who performed

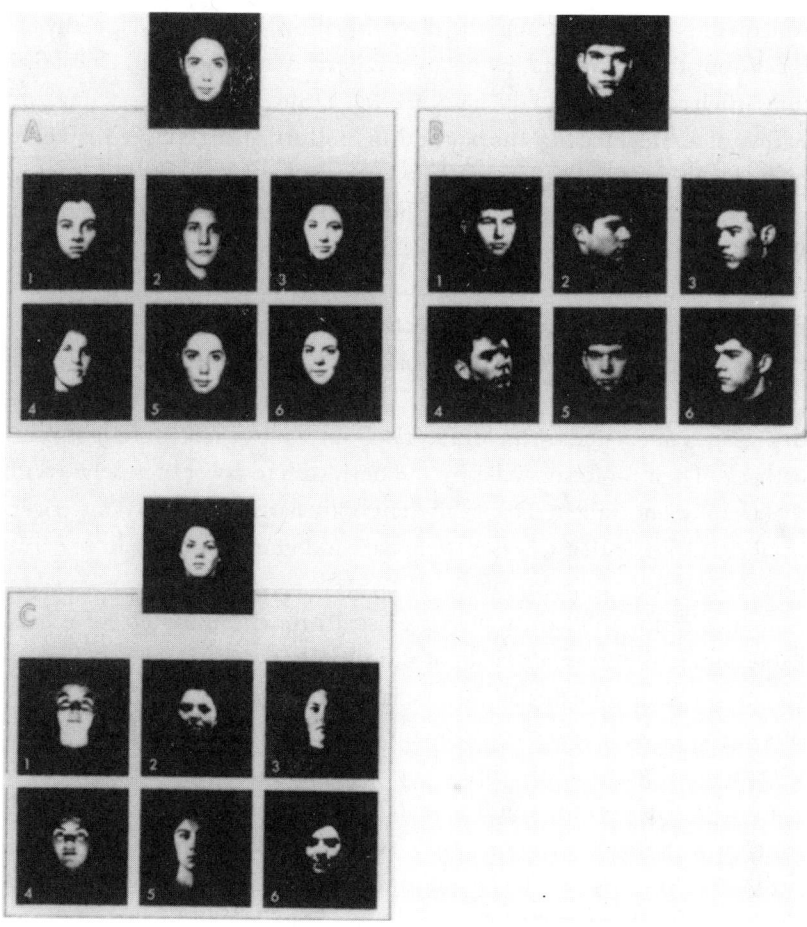

Figure 7.1
Sample items from Benton and Van Allen's (1968) Test of Facial Recognition. In part *A* the subject is required to match identical front views of faces. In part *B* the subject is required to match faces across changes in viewing angle. In part *C* the subject is required to match faces across changes in lighting.

well on tests of face matching and discrimination, but required lengthy inspections of the faces and, by his own report, relied on specific local features, such as the shape of the hairline. When the faces were shown to him with oval frames blocking the hairline, his performance dropped markedly. Newcombe points out, "Some prosopagnosic patients are reported to match faces normally. . . . Latencies, however, are not invariably measured. Where they are, they are described as abnormally slow" (p. 319). This tells us that the final scores of patients could be within normal limits when in fact their ability to perceive faces is clearly abnormal.

A huge amount of social information comes from the half square foot or so of body surface that is our face. The most obvious is individual identity. This is illustrated by the old story about the two naked students sunbathing. Their professor walks by and both rush to cover themselves with their hands, choosing to cover different body parts. The smart one covers his face, realizing that it is this body part and generally *only this body part* that enables us to be recognized.

In addition to identity, faces are usually the most immediate and reliable source of information about mood and emotional state. When assessed in prosopagnosic patients, facial expression recognition is usually impaired, but some patients maintain good emotion recognition despite impaired recognition of identity. For example, Tranel, Damasio, and Damasio (1988) report the emotion recognition ability of a series of patients, some of whom were prosopagnosic. Two of their subjects failed to recognize the identity of a single face among photographs of famous individuals as well as of their family and friends. One of these subjects was also impaired on a stringent test of facial emotion recognition, but the other performed comparably to control subjects. The perception of age and gender, two other personal characteristics of social relevance, followed the same pattern as emotion in these two cases. Young, Newcombe, de Haan, Small, and Hay (1993) found evidence of the dissociability of identity and emotional expression recognition by the performance of a large group of unilaterally brain-damaged patients.

Where a person is looking tells us what they are currently paying attention to, and this is another way in which the face provides socially relevant information. The tendency to "gaze follow," that is, look where someone else is looking, develops in infancy and can be considered a primitive form of "theory of mind," the ability to understand the mental processes of another person (Baron-Cohen, 1995). Gaze following requires the ability to discern, from slight variations in the position of the eye in the orbit, the distal location being fixated. This ability can also be impaired in prosopagnosia (Campbell, Heywood, Cowey, Regard, & Landis, 1990; unpublished data from patients L. H. and Adam). As with letter recognition in ventral simultanagnosia, the patterns of association and dissociation among face-related visual abilities suggest the existence of "specialization within specialization." Within a broad zone of visual representation optimized for encoding faces there may be more specific regions necessary for specific face-related processes such as emotion and gaze perception.

A special category of prosopagnosics are those who have been prosopagnosic since birth. We all know individuals who are poor at face recognition, and have seen their puzzlement or embarrassment when approached by a recent or casual acquaintance. In rare cases the impairment is so severe that it can be considered a congenital prosopagnosia. A few particularly severe and selective cases have been described in the literature (Bentin, Deouell, & Soroker, 1999; Duchaine, 2000; Nunn, Postma, & Pearson, 2001; Temple, 1992). The individual described by Nunn and colleagues remembers first noticing his problem at the age of seven, and reported "being unable to recognize or identify members of his own family, friends and colleagues from their faces. He also [had] difficulty recognizing actors in films, and would lose track of the plot if actors change their clothing." He was, however, normal in all other ways the authors could think to test, and had no evidence of brain damage on neurological exam or MRI. As in other cases (Bentin et al., 1999; Duchaine, 2000) there was a family history of congenital prosopagnosia, implying a genetic basis for the disorder.

These cases contrast with another individual who has been prosopagnosic since birth, due to occipitotemporal brain damage sustained as a newborn (Farah, Rabinowitz, Quinn, & Liu, 2000). This young man is mildly agnosic for objects other than faces, but is utterly unable to recognize his friends or family by their faces alone. The fact that functional object recognition systems could not take over face recognition in this case, despite the need for such recruitment prior to any experience with faces, represents an extreme lack of plasticity. Both the suggestion of heritability from the congenital cases without evidence of neurological damage, and the lack of plasticity when the relevant brain areas are damaged at birth, indicate a genetic component of visual recognition that is specific to faces.

7.4   Are Faces "Special"?

Although many prosopagnosics have some degree of difficulty recognizing objects other than faces, in many cases the deficit appears to be strikingly disproportionate for faces, with only rare difficulties with objects in everyday life. This preserved ability is sometimes used to help recognize people—for example, by a distinctive article of clothing or hair decoration. The selectivity of prosopagnosia bears directly on the issue of unity versus modularity. If faces are selectively affected, then there must be some face-specific processing component that can be damaged.

To determine whether prosopagnosia is truly selective for faces, and thus implies the existence of a specialized face module, we must determine whether faces are selectively affected merely because they are harder to recognize, or whether recognition of faces is disproportionately worse than performance on nonface objects when the difficulty of each is taken into account. In other words, we must assess prosopagnosic performance on faces and nonface objects *relative to* the difficulty of these stimuli for normal subjects. One technical difficulty encountered in such a project is that normal subjects will invariably perform nearly perfectly on both face and nonface recognition tasks. The resultant ceiling effect will mask any differences in difficulty that might exist between tasks, making it pointless to test normal subjects in the kinds of recognition tasks that have traditionally been administered to patients. With this problem in mind, researchers have devised visual recognition tasks that test learning of novel face and nonface objects. By having subjects learn to recognize specific new exemplars of faces and other types of objects, it is possible to titrate normal subjects' level of recognition performance so that it falls between ceiling and floor.

The first researchers to address this issue directly were McNeil and Warrington (1993). They studied WJ, a middle-aged professional man who became prosopagnosic following a series of strokes. After becoming prosopagnosic, WJ made a career change and went into sheep farming. He eventually came to recognize many of his sheep, although he remained unable to recognize most humans. The authors noted the potential implications of such a dissociation for the question of whether human face recognition is "special," and designed an ingenious experiment exploiting WJ's newfound career. They assembled three groups of photographs— human faces, sheep faces of the same breed kept by WJ, and sheep faces of a different breed—and attempted to teach subjects names for each face. Normal subjects performed at intermediate levels between ceiling and floor in all conditions. They performed better with the human faces than with sheep faces, even those who, like WJ, worked with sheep. In contrast, WJ performed poorly with the human faces, and performed normally with the sheep faces. These data suggest that WJ's recognition impairment does not affect the recognition of all groups of visually similar patterns, but is selective for human faces.

My colleagues and I took a similar approach, but used common objects rather than faces of another species to compare with human face recognition (Farah, Levinson, & Klein, 1995). Our subject was LH, a well-educated professional man who has been prosopagnosic since an automobile accident in college. LH is profoundly prosopagnosic, unable to reliably recognize his wife, children, or even himself in a group photograph. Yet he is highly intelligent, and seems to have little or no difficulty recognizing other types of visual patterns, such as printed words or objects. He has a degree of recognition impairment with drawings of objects, but this is less severe than his impairment with faces.

We employed a recognition memory paradigm, in which LH and control subjects first studied a set of photographs of faces and nonface objects, such as forks, chairs, and eyeglasses. Subjects were then given a larger set of photographs, and asked to make "old"/"new" judgments on them. This larger set was designed so that for each face and nonface object in the "old" set there was a highly similar item in the "new" set. Figure 7.2 shows examples of stimuli from this experiment. As a result of piloting the stimuli in advance, normal subjects performed equally well with the faces and nonface objects. In contrast, LH showed a significant performance disparity, performing worse with faces than with objects.

One could still maintain that faces possess no special status in prosopagnosia, and instead attribute the poor performance with faces to the need for within-category discrimination. Perhaps, in the words of Damasio, Damasio, and Van Hoesen (1982), "The valid dissociation is between

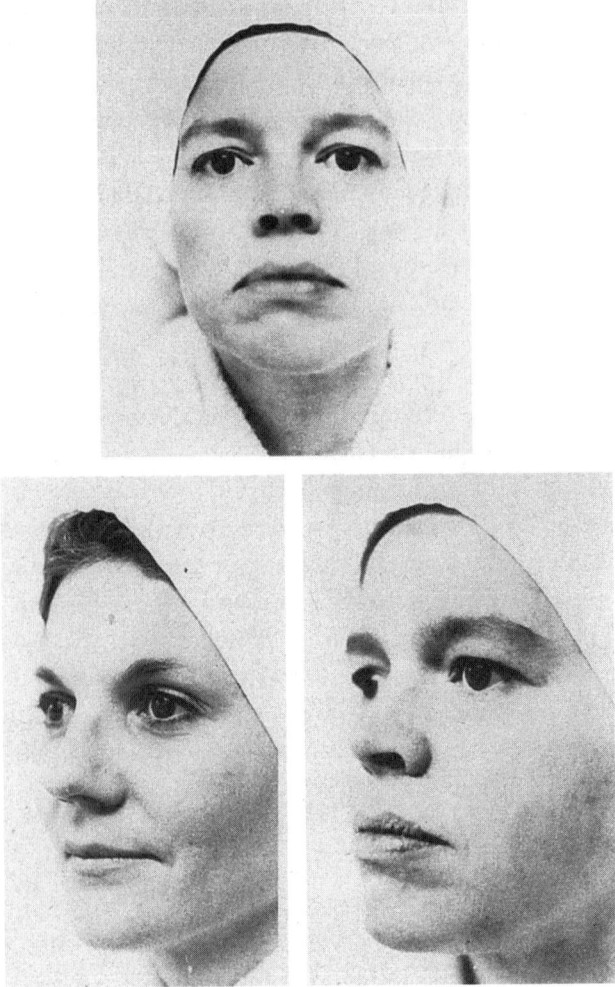

Figure 7.2
Examples of stimuli from Farah, Levinson, and Klein's (1995) experiment testing face and object recognition in prosopagnosia.

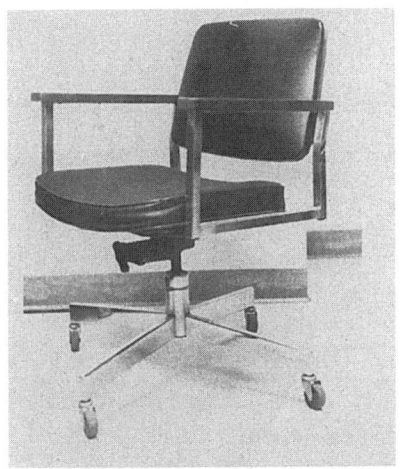

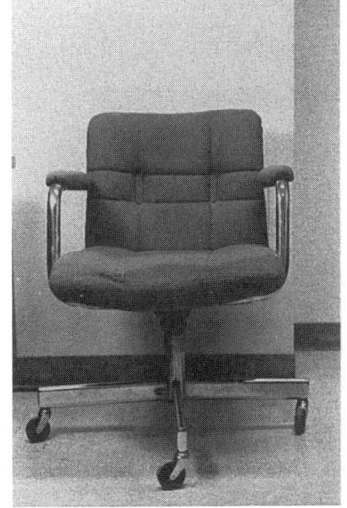
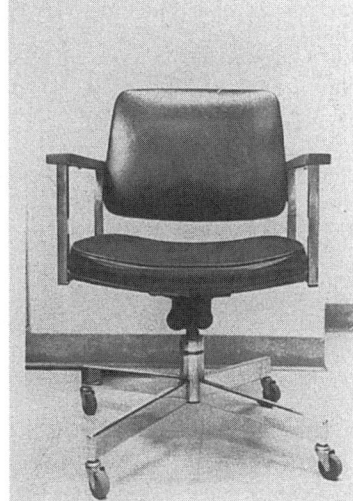

Figure 7.2
Continued

the recognition of the generic conceptual class to which the object belongs and the recognition of the historical context of a given object [i.e., the individual identity of the object] vis a vis the subject" (p. 337). To test this hypothesis directly, we carried out a second experiment in which subjects learned exemplars of the category "face" and an equivalent number of highly similar exemplars all drawn from a single nonface category, eyeglass frames. As before, LH was disproportionately impaired at face recognition relative to nonface recognition, when his performance is considered relative to normal subjects.

In a final experiment in this series, we compared LH's processing of faces to a different, and in some ways ideal, nonface control stimulus: upside-down faces (Farah, Wilson, Drain, & Tanaka, 1995). Inverted faces are are equivalent to upright faces in virtually all physical stimulus parameters, including complexity and interitem similarity. Inversion interferes with the recognition of faces more than other types of stimuli, and from this it has been inferred that inverted faces do not engage (or engage to a lesser extent) the hypothesized face-specific processing mechanisms (Valentine, 1988). We reasoned that if LH had a general recognition impairment, then he would show a normal face inversion effect. In contrast, if he had suffered damage to neural tissue implementing a specialized face recognition system, he would show an absent or attenuated face inversion effect.

LH and normal subjects were tested in a sequential matching task, in which an unfamiliar face was presented, followed by a brief interstimulus interval, followed by a second face, to which the subject responded "same" or "different." The first and second faces of a trial were always in the same orientation, and upright and inverted trials were randomly intermixed. As expected, normal subjects performed better with the upright than with the inverted faces, replicating the usual face inversion effect.

In contrast, LH was significantly more accurate with inverted faces—he showed an inverted inversion effect! This outcome was not among the alternatives we had considered. We drew two main conclusions from the inverted inversion effect. One concerns the "control structure" of visual recognition. LH's specialized face perception system was apparently contributing to his performance even though it was impaired and clearly maladaptive. This suggests that the specialized face system operates mandatorily, reminiscent of Fodor's (1983) characterization of special-purpose perceptual "modules" as engaged mandatorily by their inputs. The idea that the face system cannot be prevented from processing faces, even when damaged, also may explain why WJ was able to learn to recognize individual sheep after his strokes but could not learn to recognize human faces. The second implication concerns the selectivity of prosopagnosia. LH's disproportionate impairment on upright relative to inverted faces implies that an impairment of specialized processing mechanisms underlies his prosopagnosia.

Patients who are agnosic for objects, but not for faces, provide the other half of the double dissociation supporting specialized recognition mechanisms for faces. A number of such patients have been described in the literature (see Feinberg, Schindler, Ochoa, Kwan, & Farah, 1994, for a case series and literature review). The most detailed study of object agnosia with preserved face recognition comes from Moscovitch, Winocur, and Behrmann (1997). Their patient, CK, suffered a closed head injury resulting in severe agnosia. Despite his profound object agnosia, CK is entirely normal in his ability to recognize faces. In a test with 140 famous faces, he performed well within the range of control subjects, and even held his own with a more challenging test of famous faces photographed at different ages (e.g., Winston Churchill as a child). In one particularly enjoyable demonstration of the object-face dissociation, the experimenters showed him paintings by Archimbaldo, in which collections of objects were arranged to make faces (see figure 7.3). Whereas normal viewers quickly see both objects and faces in these pictures, CK saw only faces initially, and for most of the paintings never even noticed that there were nonface objects present!

This pattern of impairment is interesting for two reasons. First, it offers further disconfirmation of the hypothesis that prosopagnosia is just a mild disorder of a general-purpose object recognition system, with faces simply being harder to recognize than other objects. If this were true, how could it be possible for a person to do better with faces than with other objects? Second, taken in conjunction with prosopagnosia, it shows that face and object recognition are functionally independent, in that either one can continue to work without other. This rules out a single pathway with different termination points for face and nonface processing, as diagrammed in figure 7.4a, and constrains our models of the functional architecture of visual recognition to those which include parallel pathways

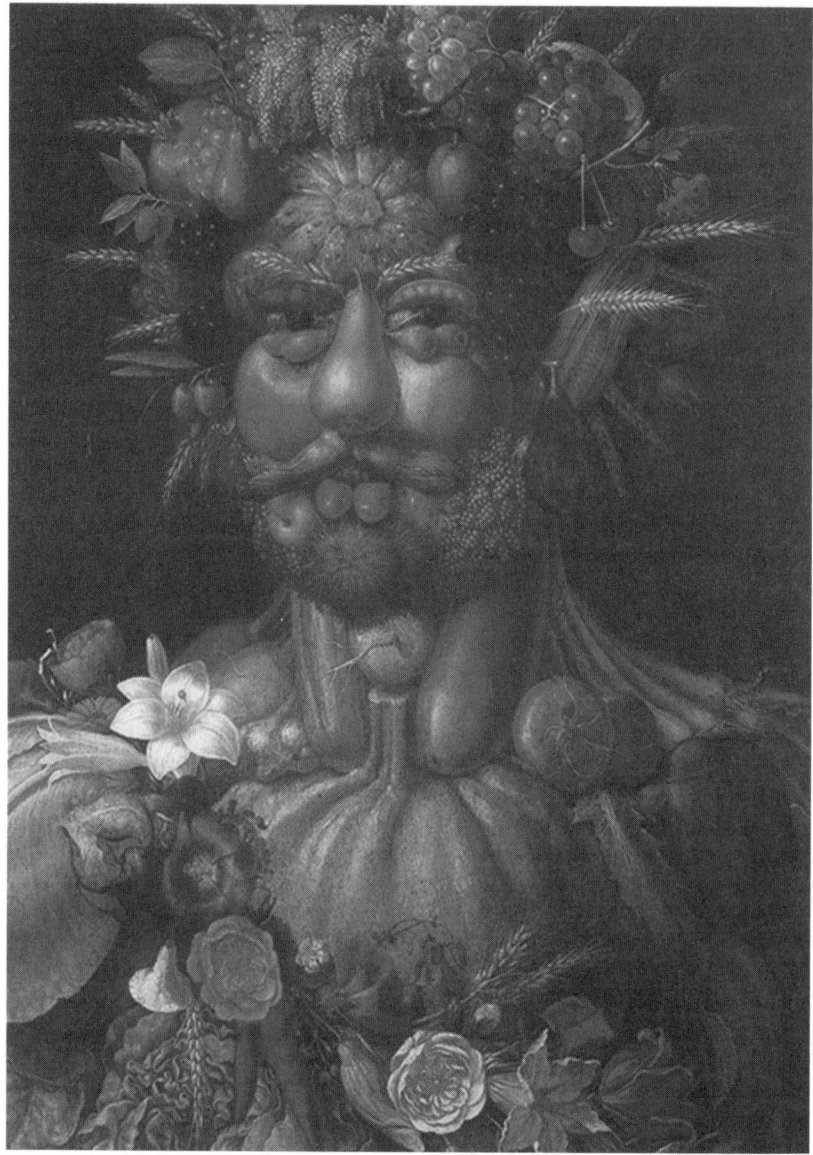

Figure 7.3
An agnosic patient with preserved face recognition studied by Moscovitch, Winocur, and
Behrmann (1997) saw only a face in this picture by Archimbaldo.

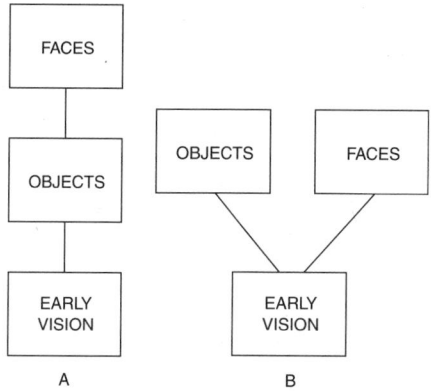

Figure 7.4
Two possible relations between an object recognition system and a specialized face recognition system.

for face and nonface object recognition, as diagrammed in figure 7.4b. This conclusion is compatible with the "two systems" hypothesis described in section 6.5.

A related double dissociation between face and object processing is instantiated by a pair of patients with material-specific amnesias. Whereas prosopagnosics are impaired at both learning new faces and recognizing previously familiar faces, consistent with damage to the substrates of face representation, my colleagues and I recently encountered someone with an even more selective impairment: following a head injury, CT became amnesic for new faces (Tippett, Miller, & Farah, 2000). In contrast, his recognition of previously familiar faces is relatively preserved, as is his learning of nonface visual objects. This pattern of performance is consistent with a disconnection between intact face representations and an intact medial temporal memory system. As such, it provides additional evidence that the anatomical substrates of face representation are distinct from the representation of other objects, since they can be selectively disconnected from the substrates of new learning.

CT's face perception was normal, and he showed an inversion effect in face matching. His learning of verbal material and of visual material other than faces was also normal. However, when given the face and eyeglass learning task, he performed similarly to LH. Additional evidence of his inability to learn faces comes from his identification of famous faces.

For people who were famous prior to CT's head injury, he performed within the range of age-matched control subjects on a forced-choice "famous/not famous" task, whereas for more recently famous individuals his performance was many standard deviations below normal. One informative exception to this is the singer Michael Jackson, who was well known before CT's injury, but whose appearance changed drastically in the years that followed. CT quickly and confidently recognized photographs of Jackson taken at about the time of his injury. However, he did not recognize a later photograph, taken the year we tested CT.

The mirror image of CT's memory impairment was described by Carlesimo, Fadda, Turriziani, Tomaiuolo, and Caltagirone (2001). Their patient, a firefighter who suffered carbon monoxide poisoning, initially appeared to be globally amnesic. He scored extremely poorly on all standard tests of memory, would repeatedly ask the same questions, and needed a list to go shopping for even a few items. Imagine the investigators' surprise when, after a single encounter at the lab with a staff member, the patient later recognized him in a different context! Subsequent testing demonstrated an island of preserved learning ability for faces in this otherwise severely amnesic patient.

In sum, the studies of prosopagnosics, object agnosics, and amnesics reviewed in this section all bear on the modularity of the functional architecture of vision. They show that faces are "special" in that they depend on neural systems which can be selectively damaged, spared, disconnected, or connected to other brain systems. Evidence from lesion reconstructions and functional neuroimaging of normal subjects, discussed in section 7.7, lends further support to the hypothesis that face processing involves at least some neural systems not used for visual object processing more generally.

7.5 Relative and Absolute Specialization

As evidence accumulated that prosopagnosia is not simply a mild general agnosia, but represents damage to a more specialized module, a different issue came to the fore. The specialized system needed for face recognition, and damaged in prosopagnosia, could be used to some degree for recognizing other types of stimuli, or it could be dedicated exclusively to face recognition. The evidence presented so far does not distinguish between these alternatives; it merely demonstrates *relatively* impaired recognition of faces without appropriate comparisons of normal and prosopagnosic non-face object recognition.

Two lines of research suggest that cerebral specialization for face recognition is not absolute, but is better described in terms of a gradient of specialization that encompasses certain nonface objects in certain task contexts. Research by De Gelder and colleagues, following up on the inverted inversion effect, provides one source of evidence (De Gelder, Bachoud-Levi, & Degos, 1998; De Gelder & Rouw, 2000). By combining a challenging object perception task, involving matching subtly differing shoes, with a face perception task, they showed an inversion effect for normal subjects with both types of stimulus, and an inverted inversion effect in prosopagnosia. They interpreted these findings in terms of the need for "configural" representation in both tasks, a conclusion that could as well be framed in terms of "holistic" representation as defined in the previous chapter.

Another source of evidence comes from the work of Gauthier, Tarr, and colleagues. They have pursued the idea that what is "special" about face recognition is the recognition of individual patterns within the general category, when the patterns share a common spatial layout and when such recognition requires extensive learning or expertise (Gauthier, Anderson, Tarr, Skudlarski, & Gore, 1997; Gauthier & Tarr, 1997; Gauthier, Williams, Tarr, & Tanaka, 1998; Gauthier, Behrmann, & Tarr, 1999). Although face recognition might be the most commonly encountered case of such ability, it need not be the only case. They have carried out a series of studies to test the hypothesis that face recognition is special only insofar as it requires subordinate classification of similarly configured shapes and is dependent on expertise. This research involves a novel class of objects called "greebles."

As can be seen in figure 7.5, greebles share a common part structure in the same way that faces do, with two "boges," a "quaff," and a "dunth." Subjects in these experiments learned names for each individual greeble. They also learned to classify the greebles by "gender" and by "family." The examples shown in figure 7.6 help to clarify what these terms mean in the context of greebles. After many hours of training, subjects became greeble experts, with fast, accurate greeble recognition and equivalent performance with subordinate (individual greeble) and basic level (gender and family) recognition.

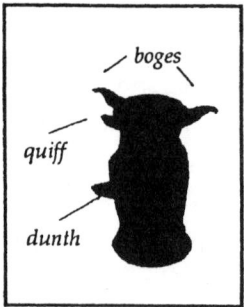

Figure 7.5
One of Gauthier and Tarr's (1997) "greebles," with key parts labeled.

GREEBLES

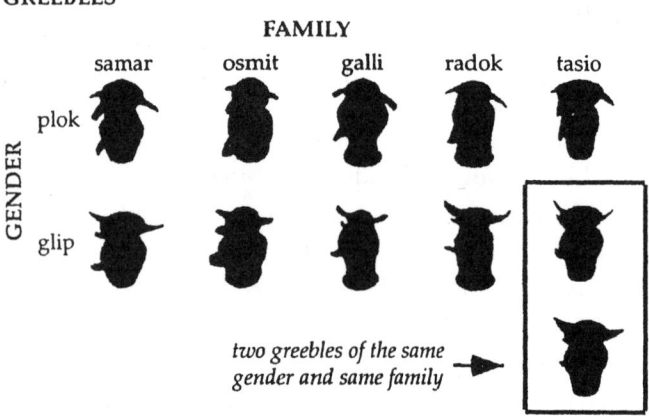

Figure 7.6
Greebles of different families and genders (Gauthier and Tarr, 1997).

Gauthier and Tarr (1997) sought to replicate, with greebles, the effects of facial context on face part discrimination that Tanaka and I found. Recall that we taught subjects new faces, and then asked them to identify a given face's eyes, nose, or mouth from a pair. With intact upright faces, but not other stimuli, subjects performed better when the pair was presented in the context of a whole face. Although greeble parts were discriminated more effectively in the context of a whole greeble, the effect was not influenced by expertise. Gauthier and Tarr did find an effect of expertise on the sensitivity of the context effects on configuration, analogous to Tanaka and Sengco's (1997) finding. In a later study, Gauthier et al. (1998) attempted to replicate a number of findings from the face recognition literature with greebles, and again obtained mixed results. The earlier finding of a whole greeble advantage for parts recognition was not replicated, and no greeble inversion effect was found. However, other purportedly face-specific effects were found with greebles, specifically the brightness inversion effect (reversing black and white makes faces and greebles hard to recognize) and the composite effect (top and bottom halves of different faces and greebles are difficult to recognize when aligned to make a whole).

Gauthier, Behrmann, and Tarr (1999) explored the recognition abilities of two prosopagnosic patients for faces, real objects, and greebles. In addition to replicating the overall disproportionate difficulty of faces for prosopagnosics shown by others, they assessed the relative difficulty of subordinate, basic, and superordinate level identification for prosopagnosics and for normal subjects. Consistent with their hypothesis that apparently face-specific processing is actually subordinate-level processing that requires expertise, they found that the patients' reaction times increased more steeply than normal as the level of categorization became more specific. The question is, are the results inconsistent with the alternative hypothesis that the system used for processing the face stimuli is not used, or is used substantially less, for processing the objects and greebles? Given that both patients had a degree of object recognition difficulty, whether resulting from the loss of the partial involvement of the system used for faces or from damage to a distinct but neighboring system, their heightened sensitivity to any sort of difficulty manipulation is not surprising.

The contribution of greeble research may be as much conceptual as empirical, since it forces us to think precisely about what we mean when we claim that "faces are 'special'." If we mean that the hypothesized face recognition system is never used in the recognition of nonface objects, then the greeble data have the potential to disconfirm the claim. If we mean that the system is specialized for a certain type of visual representation, such as the holistic representation described in chapter 6, and that its primary use is in face recognition but it may on occasion be recruited for certain other visual recognition problems, then the greeble data simply clarify the nature of the "face recognition" system's visual representations and its range of possible functions.

7.6   Covert Face Recognition in Prosopagnosia

One of the more dramatic dissociations involving prosopagnosia is the finding of preserved "covert" face recognition, that is, the ability of some patients to manifest knowledge of faces on indirect tests of recognition. The literature on covert recognition in prosopagnosia is large, dating back to the early 1980s and involving researchers from a number of different labs who were quickly drawn in by this remarkable phenomenon. Only a small sample of the relevant findings will be summarized here. One of the most widely used methods of demonstrating preserved face recognition in prosopagnosia is by the paired-associate face-name relearning task, in which patients are taught to associate the facial photographs of famous people (whom they cannot recognize) with the names of famous people. For some prosopagnosics, fewer learning trials are required when the pairing of names and faces is correct than when incorrect (e.g., Robert Redford's face with the name "Harrison Ford"). De Haan, Young, and Newcombe (1987a) showed that this pattern of performance held even when the stimulus faces were selected from among those the patient had been unable to identify in a pre-experiment stimulus screening test.

Evidence of covert recognition has also come from reaction time tasks in which the familiarity or identity of faces was found to influence processing time. In a visual identity match task with simultaneously presented pairs of faces, De Haan, Young, and Newcombe (1987a) found that a prosopagnosic patient was faster at matching pairs of previously familiar faces than unfamiliar faces, as is true of normal subjects. In contrast, he was unable to name any of the previously familiar faces.

In another RT study, De Haan, Young, and Newcombe (1987b; also 1987a) found evidence that photographs of faces could evoke covert semantic knowledge of the depicted person, despite the inability of the prosopagnosic patient to report such information about the person when tested overtly. The task was to categorize a printed name as belonging to an actor or a politician as quickly as possible. On some trials an irrelevant (i.e., to be ignored) photograph of an actor's or politician's face was simultaneously presented. Normal subjects were slower to print the names when the faces came from a different occupation category relative to a no-photograph baseline. Even though their prosopagnosic patient was severely impaired at categorizing the faces overtly as belonging to actors or politicians, he showed the same pattern of interference from different-category faces.

Prosopagnosic patients who manifest covert recognition appear to lack the subjective experience of recognition, at least for many of the faces for which they show covert recognition. These patients may occasionally recognize a face overtly, that is, assign it the correct name and express a degree of confidence that they know who the person is. However, this happens rarely, and the dissociation between covert recognition and awareness of recognition holds for many faces that they fail to identify and for which they report no sense of familiarity.

There are several competing explanations for covert recognition in prosopagnosia. The oldest is that the face recognition system is intact in these patients, but has been prevented from conveying information to other brain mechanisms necessary for conscious awareness. An explicit statement of this view comes from De Haan, Bauer, and Greve (1992), who proposed the model shown in figure 7.7. According to their model, the face-specific visual and mnemonic processing of a face (carried out

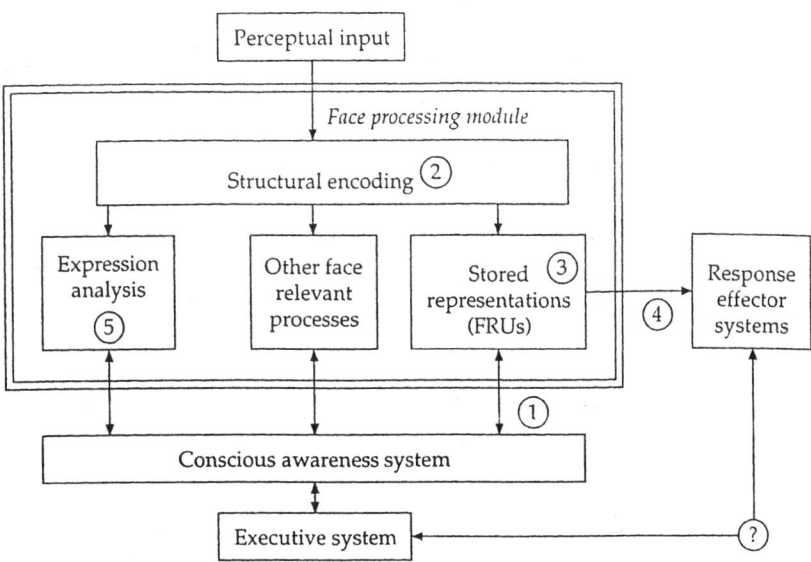

Figure 7.7
Model of face recognition used by De Haan, Bauer, and Greve (1992) to explain covert face recognition in prosopagnosia in terms of a lesion at location number 1.

within the "Face processing module") proceeds normally in covert recognition, but the results of this process cannot access the "Conscious awareness system" because of a lesion at location number 1.

Another type of explanation was put forth by Bauer (1984), who suggested that there may be two neural systems capable of face recognition, only one of which is associated with conscious awareness. According to Bauer, the ventral visual areas damaged in prosopagnosic patients are the location of normal conscious face recognition. But the dorsal visual areas are hypothesized to be capable of face recognition as well, although they do not mediate conscious recognition but, instead, affective responses to faces. Covert recognition is explained as the isolated functioning of the dorsal face system. This account also fits into the general category of consciousness as a privileged property of particular brain systems. It is analogous to theorizing about the subcortical visual system in blindsight, and the dorsal visual system in apperceptive agnosia, in that two systems are postulated that carry out related but distinct visual functions, but only one of which is endowed with conscious awareness.

Tranel and Damasio (1988) interpreted covert recognition as the normal activation of visual face representations, which is prevented by the patients' lesions from activating representations in other areas of the brain, such as representations of people's voices in auditory areas, affective valences in limbic areas, names in language areas, and so on. This idea was embodied in a computer simulation of semantic priming effects, in which covert recognition was modeled as a partial disconnection separating intact visual recognition units from the rest of the system, as shown in figure 7.8 (Burton, Young, Bruce, Johnston, & Ellis, 1991).

The foregoing explanations of covert recognition all include the assumption that visual recognition proper is intact and that the functional lesion lies outside of the visual system. A different approach to explaining covert face recognition rejects this assumption, and posits that covert recognition reflects the residual processing capabilities of a damaged, but not obliterated, visual face recognition system. Randy O'Reilly, Shaun Vecera, and I have argued that lower-quality visual information processing is needed to support performance in tests of covert recognition (e.g., to show savings in relearning, and the various RT facilitation and interference effects) relative to the quality of information processing needed to support normal overt recognition performance (e.g., naming a face, sort-

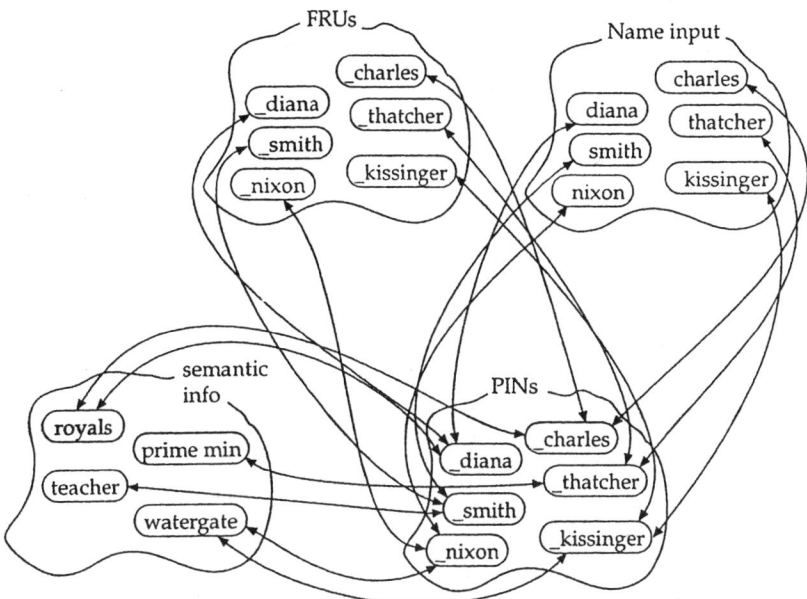

Figure 7.8
Model of face recognition used by Burton, Bruce, and Johnston (1991) to explain covert recognition in prosopagnosia in terms of a disconnection between face recognition units (FRUs) and personal identity nodes (PINs).

ing faces into those of actors and politicians; Farah, O'Reilly, & Vecera, 1993; O'Reilly & Farah, 1999). Support for this view comes from a behavioral study with normal subjects and a series of computer simulations. In the behavioral study, Wallace and Farah (1992) showed that savings in face-name relearning can be obtained with normal subjects who are trained on a set of face-name associations and then allowed for forget these associations over a six-month interval. Presumably normal forgetting does not involve the diverting of intact information from conscious awareness, but rather the degradation of representations (albeit in a different way from prosopagnosia). Probably the strongest evidence for this view, however, is computational.

Farah et al. (1993) trained a neural network, shown in figure 7.9, to associate "face" patterns with "semantic" patterns, and to associate these, in turn, with "name" patterns. We found that, at levels of damage to the face representations which led to poor or even chance performance in

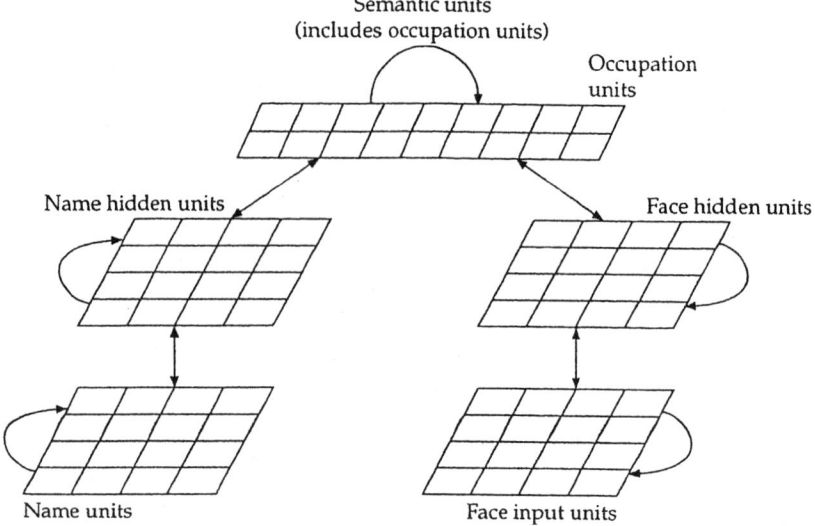

Figure 7.9

Model of face recognition used by Farah, O'Reilly, and Vecera (1993) to explain covert recognition in prosopagnosia in terms of damaged, but not obliterated, face recognition.

overt tasks such as naming (figure 7.10a) and occupation categorization, the network showed all of the behavioral covert recognition effects reviewed above: it relearned correct associations faster than it learned novel ones (figure 7.10b), it completed the visual analysis of familiar faces faster than unfamiliar faces (figure 7.10c), and it showed priming and interference from the faces on judgments about names (figure 7.10d). More recently, O'Reilly and Farah (1999) simulated several more covert recognition tasks with the same basic model.

Why should a damaged neural network support performance in this range of covert tasks when overt recognition is poor or even at chance? The answer lies in the nature of information representation and processing in distributed, interactive networks. Representations in such networks consist of patterns of activation over a set of units or neurons. These units are highly interconnected, and the extent to which the activation of one unit causes an increase or decrease in the activation of a neighboring unit depends on the "weight" of the connection between them. For the network to learn that a certain face representation goes with a certain name representation, the weights among units in the network are adjusted so that presentation of either the face pattern in the face units or the name pattern in the name units causes the corresponding other pattern to become activated. Upon presentation of the input pattern, all of the units connected with the input units will begin to change their activation in accordance with the activation value of the units to which they are connected and the weights on the connections. As activation propagates through the network, a stable pattern of activation eventually results, determined jointly by the input activation and the pattern of weights among the units of the network.

Our account of covert face recognition is based on the following key idea: The set of the weights in a network that cannot correctly associate patterns because it has never been trained (or has been trained on a different set of patterns) is different in an important way from the set of weights in a network that cannot correctly associate patterns because it has been trained on those patterns and then damaged. The first set of weights is random with respect to the associations in question, whereas the second is a subset of the necessary weights. Even if it is an inadequate subset for performing the association, it is not random; it has, "embedded" in it, some degree of knowledge of the associations. Hinton and colleagues (Hinton & Sejnowski, 1986; Hinton & Plaut, 1987) have shown that such embedded knowledge can be demonstrated when the network relearns, suggesting that the findings of savings in relearning face–name associations may be explained in this way. In general, consideration of the kinds of tests used to measure covert recognition suggest that the covert measures would be sensitive to this embedded knowledge. The most obvious example is that a damaged network would be expected to relearn associations which it previously knew faster than novel associations because of the nonrandom starting weights as shown in figure 7.10b. Less obvious, the network would settle faster when given previously learned inputs than novel inputs (figure 7.10c), because the residual weights come from a set designed to create a stable pattern from that input. Finally, to the extent that the weights continue to activate partial and subthreshold patterns over the nondamaged units in association with the input, these resultant patterns could prime (i.e., contribute toward) the activation of patterns by intact routes (figure 7.10d).

The general implication of these ideas is that as a neural network is increasingly damaged, there will be a window of damage in which overt

(a)

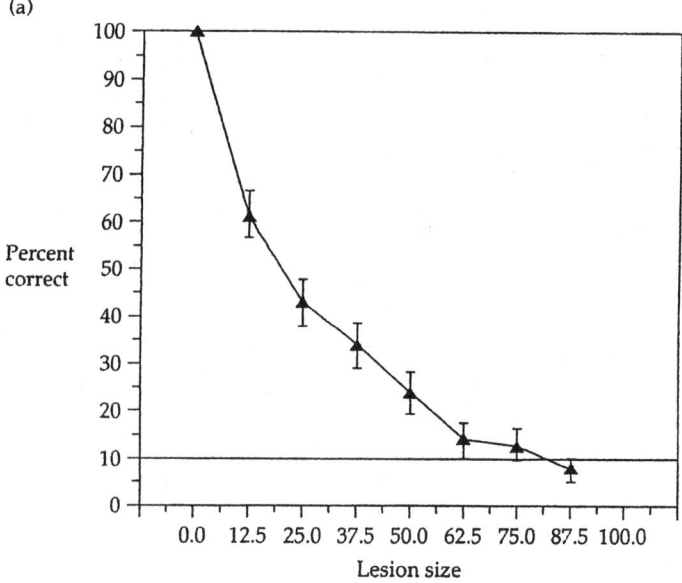

(b)

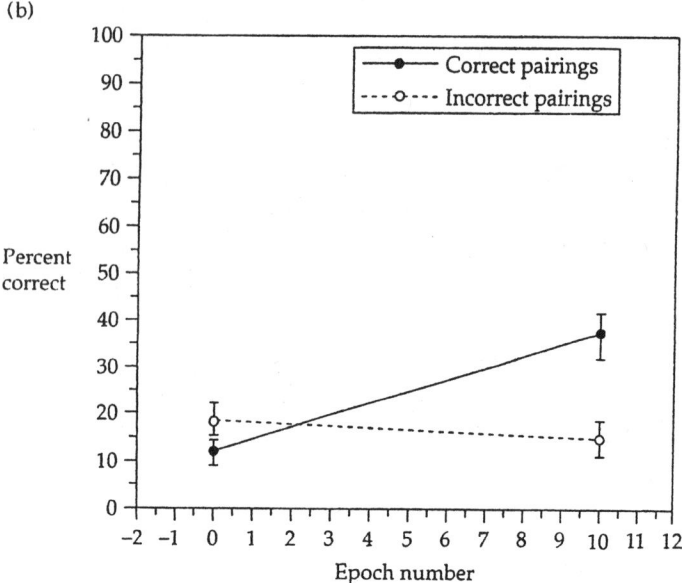

Figure 7.10

Representative results of simulations of different covert recognition phenomena, from the model shown in figure 7.9.

(c)

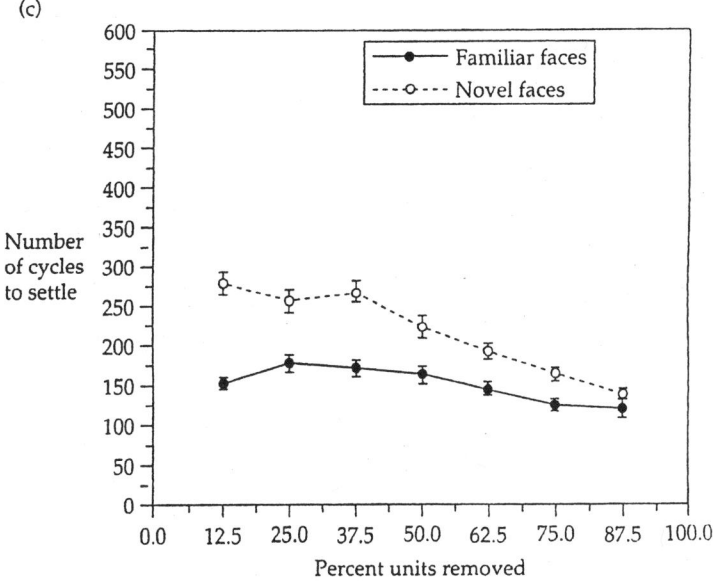

(d)

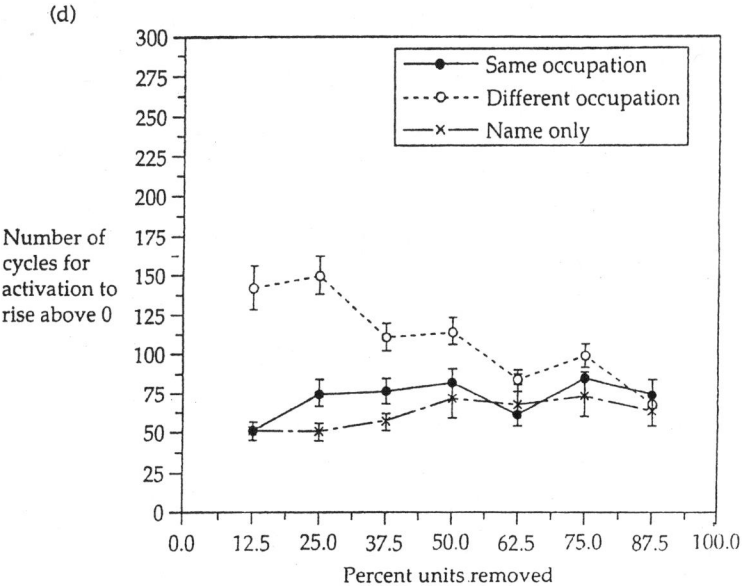

associations between patterns (e.g., faces and names) would be extremely poor while the kinds of performance measures tapped by the covert tasks might remain at high levels.

7.7   Neuropathology of Prosopagnosia

The lesions of prosopagnosia have received much attention. All writers agree that a right hemisphere lesion is necessary. Discussion has focused on the intrahemispheric location of the right hemisphere lesion and on the necessity for a second, left hemisphere lesion. In an early attempt at generalization, Meadows (1974) reviewed the clinical case literature on prosopagnosia and used visual field defects and autopsy reports to infer the distribution of lesion sites. The almost invariable finding of a left superior quadrananopia indicated that the right inferior occipitotemporal was critical, and the frequent finding of smaller field defects on the right suggested a tendency for bilateral damage. These conclusions were supported by the findings in those cases that came to autopsy. Damasio, Damasio, and Van Hoesen (1982) arrived at similar conclusions, emphasizing the need for bilateral lesions.

A revision of this view was urged by DeRenzi, Perani, Carlesimo, Silveri, and Fazio (1994), who reviewed much of the same case material, along with more recent cases and data from living patients whose brain damage was mapped using both structural MRI and PET. Their findings supported the ventral, occipitotemporal localization of face recognition, but called for a revision of the idea that bilateral lesions are necessary. Some patients became prosopagnosic after unilateral right hemisphere damage. The possibility of hidden left hemisphere dysfunction in these cases was reduced by the finding of normal metabolic activity in the left hemisphere by PET scan. De Renzi et al. conclude that there is a spectrum of hemispheric specialization for face recognition in normal right-handed adults. Although the right hemisphere may be relatively better at face recognition than the left, most people have a degree of face recognition ability in both hemispheres. Nevertheless, in a minority of cases, face recognition is so focally represented in the right hemisphere that a unilateral lesion will lead to prosopagnosia.

The localization of face recognition has also been the focus of extensive research using functional neuroimaging, with the conclusions of

the two approaches in good agreement with one another. Early comparisons of face recognition with other visual-spatial tasks confirmed the occipitotemporal localization inferred from lesion studies (e.g., Haxby et al.,
1991). As experimental designs were refined and more specific stimulus
contrasts were included to isolate face-specific regions (for example, contrasting faces with objects, houses, body parts, and even inverted faces),
the "fusiform face area" (FFA) became more focally and reliably localized
(e.g., Haxby et al., 1999; Kanwisher, Tong, & Nakayama, 1998; Kanwisher, McDermott, & Chun, 1997; Kanwisher, Stanley, & Harris, 1999;
McCarthy, Puce, Gore, & Allison, 1997). Figure 7.11 shows the location
of the FFA in two subjects, on the basis of an fMRI experiment with alternating blocks of faces, houses and objects (Tong, Nakayama, Moscovitch, Weinrib, & Kanwisher, 2000). A recent report of prosopagnosia
following a small hematoma affecting the FFA demonstrates the conver-
gence of the lesion and functional imaging approaches to the anatomy of
face recognition (Wada & Yamamoto, 2001).

7.8   Topographic Agnosia: A Case Description

Like faces, scenes and landmarks are visual stimuli with great importance
to our survival. Hunting, gathering, seeking mates, and seeking refuge all
require knowledge of one's location within the environment, which
scenes and landmarks provide. It is probably no coincidence that half of
the paintings in any museum gallery are either portraits or landscapes.

Recognition of scenes and landmarks is sometimes impaired in conjunction with prosopagnosia, but the two also occur in isolation. A particularly pure case of topographic agnosia was described by Whitely and
Warrington (1978). Following a severe head injury incurred in a motor
vehicle accident, a forty-six-year-old workman recovered most of his premorbid abilities except for a specific problem with visual recognition.

His present complaint, four years after the accident, is of a failure to recognize
buildings, streets, and other landmarks, which incapacitates him to the extent that
he gets lost in familiar surroundings. He describes looking at a building, being
able to see and describe it clearly, yet if he looks away and looks back again, it looks
different as though someone had put another unfamiliar building in its place. The
street in which he lives seems unfamiliar, and each day he might be going along

Axial   Coronal

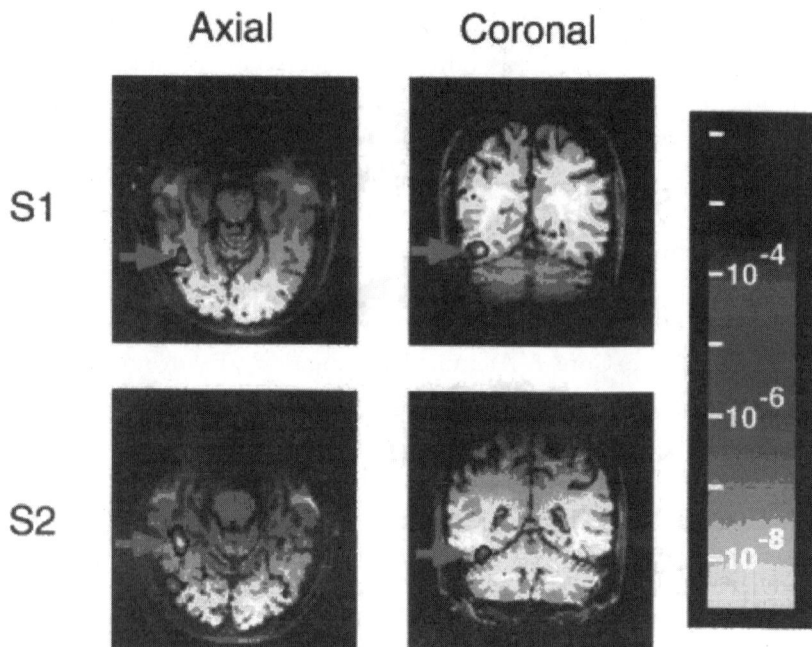

Figure 7.11
The location of the fusiform face area in two subjects, on the basis of an fMRI experiment with alternating blocks of faces, houses and objects (Tong et al., 2000).

it as for the first time. He recognizes his own house by the number, or by his car when parked at the door.

He complains of considerable difficulty in getting about, and says that learning new routes presents a real problem. He can, however, use a map easily and follow verbal instructions. He relies heavily on street names, station names, and house numbers.

Apart from these topographical difficulties, he reports only a minor degree of difficulty in recognizing people's faces, especially people he has met recently, and a minor degree of nonspecific forgetfulness. He is, nevertheless, able to read a book and follow a film or play without difficulty. He has noticed no difficulty in writing, drawing, or making scale plans.

Whitely and Warrington administered a wide range of perception and memory tests without finding any more general impairments that might have been responsible for this patient's topographic agnosia. They assessed his ability to perceive buildings with a matching task in which pairs of photographs of buildings, taken from different angles, were placed side by side and judged to be the same or different buildings. Although the authors conclude from the patient's perfect performance on this task that his perception of buildings is normal, the task does allow piecemeal visual comparison and may therefore overestimate his abilities. In contrast, he performed below the worst control subject in learning to recognize new buildings and at the low end of the normal range in recognizing famous city landmarks, consistent with his difficulty in learning his way around new locales and recognizing his own street and home.

7.9   General Characteristics of Topographic Agnosia and Related Disorders

There are a small number of similar cases in the literature. Some have prosopagnosia in addition to topographic agnosia, such as Pallis's (1955) case that was excerpted in section 7.2, and those of Cole and Perez-Cruet (1964) and Landis, Cummings, Benson and Palmer (1986, cases 2 and 4). In other cases, the topographic agnosia is an isolated visual recognition deficit: Incisa della Rocchetta, Cippolotti, and Warrington (1996), Hecaen, Tzortzis, and Rondot (1980), and Landis et al. (1986, cases 1 and 3). The impairment is appropriately grouped with disorders of visual recognition rather than of spatial cognition, in that the patients' spatial abilities are preserved. Indeed, it is typically reported that patients develop a heavy dependence on their preserved spatial abilities to find their way around the environment and are able to use maps (Hecaen et al., 1980; Icisa della Rocchetta et al., 1996; Landis et al., 1986, cases 1 and 2; Whitely & Warrington, 1978). Because of the specificity of the recognition impairment, patients are able to recognize common objects, and also report using these objects to help them orient themselves—for example, exterior objects such as mailboxes, water fountains, phone booths, palm trees, or a certain style of lettering, and interior objects such as the ward phonograph or a certain color wall (examples from the cases of Landis et al., 1986). New learning of scenes and landmarks is dramatically impaired, along with recognition of personally familiar locales and, in all but Whitely and Warrington's case, famous landmarks. Incisa della Rocchetta et al. separately tested the recognition of country landscapes, devoid of human constructions, and city scapes, and found both severely impaired.

Topographic agnosia should be distinguished from other disorders affecting orientation within the large-scale environment. Aguirre and D'Esposito (1999) offer a useful taxonomy of impairments in the realm of navigation and way-finding. Of the four categories in their taxonomy, two concern purely spatial processing impairments. More likely to be confused are the remaining two, the disorder of topographic agnosia described here and a disorder of new learning that affects both visual and spatial aspects of the environment (e.g., Epstein et al., 2001; Habib & Sirigu, 1987; Katayama, Takahashi, Ogawara, & Hattori, 1999). Patients with the latter disorder can recognize premorbidly familiar locales, but have difficulty learning both the features and the layout of new environments.

7.10   Neuropathology of Topographic Agnosia

Topographic agnosia most commonly follows right or bilateral posterior artery infarction, although Whitely and Warrington's patient suffered a head injury and Incisa della Rocchetta's patient had diffuse damage due to small vessel ischemic disease. When focal lesions can be visualized, they are similar to those of prosopagnosia, affecting inferior medial occipito-temporal cortex, including the fusiform and lingual gyri and in some cases extending into the parahippocampal gyrus, either on the right side or bilaterally. Functional neuroimaging has provided converging evidence for topography-specific representations in the lingual and parahippocampal gyri (Aguirre, Zarahn, & D'Esposito, 1998; Epstein & Kanwisher, 1998), consistent with the lesions just described.

Chapter 8

Optic Aphasia

8.1 Optic Aphasia: A Case Description

Optic aphasia is a puzzling disorder in which patients cannot name visually presented objects, despite demonstrating good visual recognition nonverbally (e.g., by pantomiming the use of a seen object or sorting semantically related objects together) and good naming (e.g., by naming palpated objects or objects they hear described verbally). Given that they can get from vision to semantics (intact visual recognition) and from semantics to naming (intact object naming of nonvisual inputs), one would expect them to be able to name visually presented objects.

One of the most thoroughly studied cases of optic aphasia was described by Lhermitte and Beauvois (1973). Their subject, Jules F, suffered a posterior left hemisphere stroke, with some amnesia, pure alexia, and mild constructional apraxia and color vision deficit. Although he made relatively few errors in naming objects from verbal definition (5/125), or from their characteristic noises or their feel in his hand (1/25 and 11/120, respectively), he made a large number of errors (35/130) in naming visually presented objects and pictures. Although he performed well on a task of pointing to a visual stimulus depicting a spoken name, the authors point out that the choice set of possible responses in this task is much smaller than in the naming tasks just described, suggesting that performance in this task may not be truly better than in naming visually presented stimuli when overall difficulty is accounted for. They also point out that when the named item was absent, Jules pointed to incorrect choices that were semantically related to the word, apparently without any awareness that the correct choice was missing.

Based on his naming performance in different modalities, it is clear that Jules F. is not simply anomic, but has a specific problem naming visual stimuli. However, the data so far are consistent with his being a visual agnosic, or even blind. The second critical element for classifying him as an optic aphasic is the ability to demonstrate recognition of visually presented stimuli by means other than naming. A common nonverbal means of communicating recognition, often used spontaneously by patients like Jules F, is to gesture the use of the object in pantomime. Lhermitte and Beauvois presented the patient with 100 pictures of common objects, and report that whenever he mimed the use of an object, he did so correctly, even when he misnamed the object. For example, when shown a picture of a boot, he mimed pulling on a boot but called it a hat. Thus, the authors conclude that the visual naming deficit cannot be attributed to agnosia. Consistent with this is their observation that the patient had no trouble interacting with the visual world in everyday life. They do mention occasional agnosialike behavior with certain complex objects: he can sometimes copy or describe the appearance of a stimulus accurately without being able to identify it by any means.

The patient's errors in naming visual stimuli seemed to be mainly semantic in nature, with many perseverations of responses from previous trials. Visual errors without semantic similarity were reported to be relatively rare, although many errors showed both visual and semantic similarity to the correct response. When given unlimited time to name a visual stimulus, Jules F would generally home in on the correct name. However, several attempts were often necessary, as is evident in the following protocol (Lhermitte and Beauvois, 1973, pp. 706–707):

A grasshopper: "a cricket, not a cricket, a grasshopper."

A mussel: "it looks like 2 snails, 2 slugs, it is a shellfish, not an oyster, it should be mussels then."

A bus: "a wagon . . . a public transport since there is a back door . . . a stagecoach . . . it would be . . . no . . . a city cab . . . not a cab but a city bus."

A window-blind: "A parasol, metallic curtain rods . . . the cloth roof . . . surrounding sails . . . it could be a parasol . . . there are rods, but isn't it a shelter? A window-blind."

An aquarium: "A bird cage, unless it is a pot for flowers, a container, a tank, the four aspects . . . the walls made of glass or wood . . . it could be an aquarium if it is made of glass."

A medieval crown: [a preceding picture had correctly been named "basket"] "a kind of foot of metallic basket, a basket for flowers, a basket for a table . . . it cannot be a basket for decoration on a table . . . it is not a decoration, I do not know what it could be. . . . A basket with 4 feet, no with 4 crossed hoops . . . it cannot be worn as clothing, it would be a hat. It would be a very fancy hat to look like that."

In order to determine whether objects were misnamed because they were misperceived, or whether the naming errors were generated after an adequate perceptual analysis was complete, Lhermitte and Beauvois asked the subject to draw what he had seen and what he had named on trials in which objects were misnamed. When asked to draw what he had seen, he invariably drew a recognizable picture of the stimulus, which was distinguishable from his drawing of the named item. For example, on one trial the stimulus was a tree and Jules F said, "it's a house with a straw roof," a perseveration from a previous trial in which a house was shown. When requested to draw what he had seen, he drew a tree, insisting all the while that he was drawing a "straw roof," and when requested to draw a house, he produced a good drawing of a house. Lhermitte and Beauvois conclude that processing within the visual system is roughly intact and cannot be the cause of the errors in visual naming. Another observation that is consistent with this conclusion comes from testing with tachistoscopic stimulus presentations. Jules F would often continue to search for and home in on the correct name for a picture long after the picture had disappeared, as if he had gotten sufficient visual information in the brief presentation and the laborious part of the visual naming process was postvisual.

8.2 General Characteristics of Optic Aphasia

A number of other cases of optic aphasia have been described in the literature, including Assal and Regli (1980); Campbell and Manning (1996); Chanoine, Ferreira, Demonet, Nespoulous, and Poncet (1998); Coslett and Saffran (1989, 1992); Gil, Pluchon, Toullat, Michenau, Rogez, and Lefevre (1985); Goldenberg and Karlbauer (1998); Hillis and Caramazza (1995); Larrabee et al. (1985, case 2); Poeck (1984); Riddoch and Humphreys (1987b); and Spreen, Benton, and Van Allen (1966). These cases show a strong similarity to that of Lhermitte and Beauvois in several respects. Naming is normal or relatively unimpaired for objects presented in the tactile modality and for sounds, as well as to spoken definition.

Reading, as well as naming of visually presented objects and pictures, is invariably poor. Like the case of Lhermitte and Beauvois, five of these patients can often demonstrate their recognition by gesturing appropriately to a visual stimulus (Coslett & Saffran, 1992; Gil et al., 1985; Goldenberg & Karlbauer, 1998; Hillis & Caramazza, 1995; Riddoch & Humphreys, 1987b). In two other cases, the patients could not be discouraged from naming the objects before making their gestures, and the gestures would then be made for the named object rather than for the visually presented object (Coslett & Saffran, 1989; Larrabee et al., 1985).

The errors of some patients frequently bear no obvious relation to the target name, but for other patients such errors are rare. Perseverations are common in all cases. When naming errors can be classified in terms of their relation to the target word, they are predominantly semantic. For example, "vines" for a trellis (Coslett & Saffran, 1989) or "cigarette lighter" for lamp (Gil et al., 1985). Visual errors bearing no semantic relationship to the stimulus were relatively rare in these cases, although they were noted to occur occasionally in many cases (Coslett & Saffran, 1989; Gil et al., 1985; Goldenberg & Karlbauer, 1998; Hillis & Caramazza, 1995; Lhermitte & Beauvois, 1973; Riddoch & Humpreys, 1987b). In general, visual perception seems intact. Hillis and Caramazza (1995) assessed object perception in a number of ways, including the delayed copying task described in the earlier excerpt. Like the patient of Lhermitte and Beauvois, this patient invariably drew the correct picture, while in each case naming it incorrectly! Also consistent with intact perception, the visual quality of the stimulus has little or no effect on these patients' naming performance: When reported separately, the naming of objects, photographs, and drawings shows little or no difference (Gil et al., 1985; Larrabee et al., 1985; Lhermitte & Beauvois, 1973; Poeck, 1984; Riddoch & Humphreys, 1987b).

Although early descriptions of optic aphasia reported visual recognition to be intact, more recent studies have used more stringent tests of patients' comprehension of visual stimuli, and obtained mixed results. On the one hand, several types of nonverbal task have provided evidence of visual recognition by optic aphasic patients: Success in pantomiming the use of a visually presented object demonstrates access to semantics from vision, as does normal or near-normal performance in classification tasks that require semantically related visual stimuli to be grouped together. For example, given a set of pictures of furniture, vehicles, and animals, the subject is to put the items in the same categories together. Optic aphasic patients do well in such tasks (Assal & Regli, 1980; Chanoine et al., 1998; Coslett & Saffran, 1989; Hillis & Caramazza, 1995; Riddoch & Humphreys, 1987b). On the other hand, classification tasks requiring finer distinctions are difficult for these patients (Chanoine et al., 1998; Gil et al., 1985; Goldenberg & Karlbauer, 1998; Hillis & Caramazza, 1995; Riddoch & Humphreys, 1987b). For example, whereas Chanoine's patient performed perfectly when fairly general semantic category information was tested (putting *envelope* with one of the following three items: *stamp, cube* and *stairs*), he performed at chance when subtler information is required (putting *palm tree* with *pyramid* rather than *fir tree*).

Why do optic aphasics fail these more difficult tests of vision-to-semantic processing? Are they really impaired in understanding the meaning of visually presented stimuli, and is this what underlies their visual naming impairment? Much rides on the answers to these questions, because they imply entirely different models of the optic aphasic impairment and, by extension, normal visual naming. Although it is possible that optic aphasics are truly unable to derive a normal amount of semantic information from the visual appearance of objects, there are at least two reasons to question that conclusion. First, the everyday behavior of optic aphasic patients does not suggest impaired access to semantics from vision. In contrast, patients with semantic memory impairments (to be discussed in the next section) and visual agnosic patients are noticeably handicapped in real life by their inability to understand what they see. Furthermore, even ostensibly nonverbal tasks benefit from verbal mediation, and this seems especially true when irrelevant visual similarities and cross–cutting categorical associations are present. The unavailability of verbal codes when classifying visual stimuli, or the intrusion of inappropriate verbal codes, rather than the unavailability of semantic information per se, may underlie the poor performance of optic aphasic patients on stringent semantic tasks.

8.3   Neuropathology of Optic Aphasia

The neuropathology of optic aphasia shows a fair degree of uniformity. All cases appear to have unilateral left posterior lesions; in cases with sufficient localizing evidence, the damage seems to include the occipital cortex and white matter. On the basis of their literature review, Schnider, Benson, and Scharre (1994) suggest that damage to the splenium (the most posterior portion of the corpus callosum) is invariably present, and distinguishes the lesions of optic aphasia from those of visual object agnosia after unilateral left hemisphere damage.

8.4 Relation Between Optic Aphasia and Associative Visual Agnosia

Associative agnosics and optic aphasics share many characteristics. They cannot name visually presented stimuli, even though their naming of tactile and auditory stimuli is relatively unimpaired. In addition, both types of patients demonstrate apparently good elementary visual perception, as measured by their ability to copy drawings that they cannot name and describe the visual appearance of objects. For this reason, the distinction between them has not always been clearly drawn. For example, Ferro and Santos (1984) published a detailed report titled "Associative Visual Agnosia: A Case Study," in which they reported that the patient could almost always pantomime the use of an object if he failed to name it (p. 125), and that his sorting of visually presented objects was reasonably good (p. 129: 80 percent correct for objects) and not very different from his performance on the analogous test with spoken words rather than visual stimuli (p. 127: 90 percent correct). His naming errors were most often perseverations, and more often anomic or semantic than visual (p. 126). His ability to name pictures was insensitive to perceptual factors such as size and inspection time (p. 126). The confusion between associative agnosia and optic aphasia is not unique to this case. Indeed the famous case of Lissauer (1890), which prompted him to draw the apperceptive/associative distinction, appears to have had a mixture of agnosia and optic aphasia, given the patient's frequent semantic errors and perseverations.

Geschwind (1965) classified associative agnosia and optic aphasia as a single syndrome; Bauer and Rubens (1985) and Kertesz (1987) suggested that they differ only in degree rather than in kind; and Davidoff and De Bleser (1993) drew a more qualitative distinction while nevertheless highlighting the commonality of impaired visual naming. Although there may indeed be underlying continuities between agnosia, optic aphasia, and a third disorder, anomia (see figure 8.7), there are also multiple and intercorrelated distinctive characteristics that compel even an avid "lumper" to split them into separate categories.

The most obvious difference is the ability of optic aphasics to derive at least a degree of semantic information from the visual appearance of an object, as shown by their pantomime and classification performance. Related to this difference is the impact of the disorder on everyday life: associative agnosics are often noted to be handicapped by an inability to recognize people, common objects, and locales, whereas no such difficulties are faced by optic aphasics. Associative agnosics show tremendous sensitivity to the visual quality of the stimulus, identifying real objects more accurately than photographs and photographs more accurately than drawings, and identifying visual stimuli better at long exposure durations than at short ones, whereas optic aphasics are insensitive to this task dimension. The nature of the errors made by these two kinds of patients differs as well: visual errors predominate in associative agnosia, whereas semantic errors and perseverations predominate in optic aphasia. Note that these differences are not differences in degree, such that optic aphasics have the same characteristics as agnosics but in milder form. Optic aphasics show *more* perseveration and semantic errors than associative agnosics. At roughly equivalent levels of naming peformance, associative agnosics are affected by visual stimulus quality, whereas optic aphasics are not. In summary, there are several characteristics that occur with great consistency within only one or the other of these groups of patients. This is inconsistent with a single disorder varying along a single dimension of severity. We will return to the relation between optic aphasia and associative visual agnosia in the next section, in the context of an explanation for optic aphasia.

8.5   Explaining Optic Aphasia: A Challenge for Conventional Cognitive Theory

What sorts of representations and processes underlie the normal ability to name visual stimuli, and which of these has been damaged in optic aphasia? At first glance the answer seems perfectly obvious: optic aphasia appears to be a cut-and-dried case of a disconnection syndrome, in which intact vision centers are separated from intact naming centers. However, on closer examination of the abilities and deficits of these patients, optic aphasia poses a serious paradox that is difficult to dispel within the framework of conventional models of visual naming.

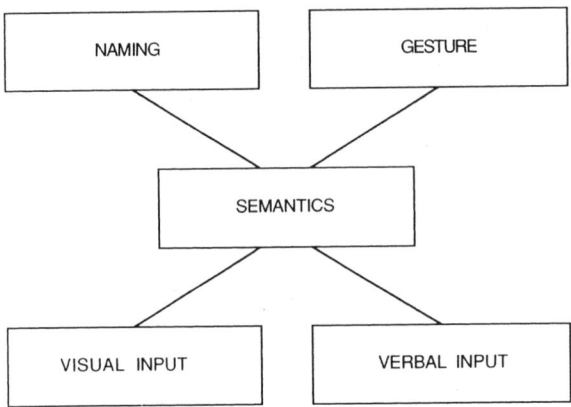

Figure 8.1
A simplified but uncontroversial model of the systems underlying the recognition of visual and nonvisual stimuli, with verbal and nonverbal responses.

It is generally assumed that the functional architecture underlying visual naming must include three major components—vision, semantics, and naming, related to one another as shown in figure 8.1. Exactly what these vision, semantics, and naming mean in this context may not be entirely clear, but the gist of such an account must surely be correct in the following sense. In order to name a visually presented object, I must see it clearly enough to be able to access some semantic information about it (i.e., to know what it is), and once I know what it is, I must then retrieve and produce its name. Surprisingly, there is no part of this model that can be damaged to produce optic aphasia. Given that optic aphasics can gesture appropriately to visual stimuli they cannot name, and correctly sort or match visual stimuli according to semantic attributes, then their impairment cannot lie anywhere in vision, semantics, or the path between the two. Given that they can supply the appropriate name to verbal definitions, sounds, and palpated objects, then their impairment cannot lie anywhere in semantics, naming operations, or the path between the two. Note that all possible loci for damage in this simple model of visual naming have just been eliminated!

In order to account for optic aphasia, the model presented in figure 8.1 has been revised in various ways. The earliest attempt to explain optic aphasia in terms of a model of normal processing was by Ratcliff and Newcombe (1982), later elaborated by Davidoff and De Bleser (1993).

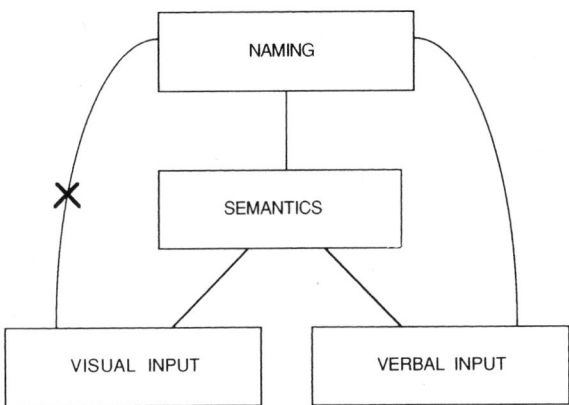

Figure 8.2
A cognitive architecture for explaining optic aphasia, with a direct route from vision to naming, based on the ideas of Ratcliff and Newcombe (1982) and Davidoff and De Blesser (1993).

They recognized the paradoxical nature of the disorder and suggested that the least unappealing solution is to postulate a direct route from vision to naming. According to this model, shown in figure 8.2 in addition to semantically mediated object naming, there is also a nonsemantic route whereby specific visual percepts can evoke their corresponding names directly. In normal visual naming, the two routes are used in parallel and together produce accurate, reliable naming. In optic aphasia, the direct route has been interrupted, and the loss of this redundancy decreases the reliability of the system. Although the basic phenomena of optic aphasia are accounted for by adding a separately lesionable route from vision to language, there is no independent support for the existence of such a route.

Another way to account for optic aphasia is to postulate multiple semantic systems, each associated with a different modality. Beauvois (1982) proposed that optic aphasia can be explained as a disconnection between visual and verbal semantics, as shown in figure 8.3. Although she did not define these two terms explicitly, her discussion of them implies that visual semantics consists of visual information about objects, which can be accessed by stimuli of any modality, and verbal semantics consists of verbal associations and abstract properties of objects that cannot be visualized or represented concretely in any particular modality, also accessible by stimuli of any modality. This subdivision of semantics by modality works

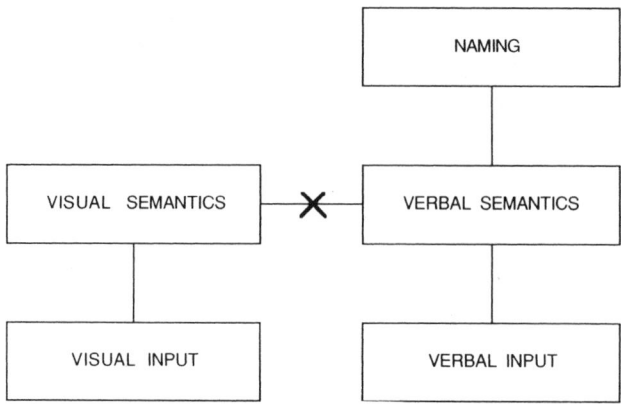

Figure 8.3
A cognitive architecture for explaining optic aphasia with separate modality-specific semantic systems, based on the ideas of Beauvois (1982).

well to explain the phenomena described by Beauvois and Saillant (1985) in a case of "optic aphasia for colors." Although Beauvois's idea of modality-specific semantic systems does an excellent job of accounting for the behavior of her patient with color tasks, it does not account well for the broader range of phenomena that constitute the syndrome of optic aphasia. For example, the largely preserved ability of optic aphasics to sort visually dissimilar objects into superordinate categories and to match visually presented objects based on function (e.g., a button and a zipper) cannot be explained in this. One could revise the modality-specific semantics account to account for optic aphasic by defining the "visual semantics" of figure 8.3 as a complete store of general knowledge—including object function, categorical relations with superordinate concepts, and so on— that is accessed only by visually presented stimuli. However, the notion that we have multiple "copies" of our entire stock of semantic knowledge, one for each modality of stimulus presentation, seems just as ad hoc as the direct route from vision to language.

Riddoch and Humphreys (1987b) suggest an interpretation of optic aphasia according to which semantics is a unitary entity, and place the processing breakdown between vision and semantics, as shown in Figure 8.4. Accordingly, they classify optic aphasia as a kind of agnosia, which they call "semantic access agnosia," because vision is normal but there is diffi-

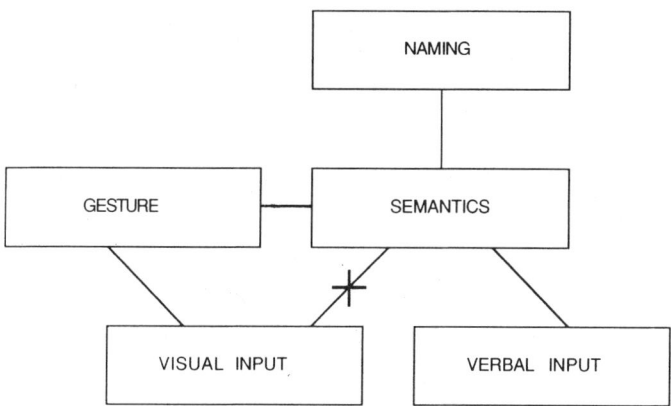

Figure 8.4

A cognitive architecture for explaining optic aphasia as a disconnection between vision and semantics, based on the ideas of Riddoch and Humphreys (1986).

culty accessing semantic information with the products of visual perception. This conception of optic aphasia coincides with the traditional conception of associative agnosia as "normal perception, stripped of its meaning." The question is, how well does this conception of optic aphasia account for the abilities and deficits of optic aphasics? How, for example, can it be squared with the successful gesturing of many of these patients in response to a visual stimulus?

Riddoch and Humphreys argue that gesturing is a misleading measure of semantic access for two reasons: First, gestures are inherently less precise than names and are therefore a less precise means of testing comprehension. To use an example provided by Ratcliff and Newcombe (1982), the gestures for a sock and a shoe are virtually identical, whereas the names are highly discriminable and a patient who said "sock" when shown a shoe would be considered to have made a semantic error. Although this is true, it cannot alone account for the difference in gesturing and naming performance in optic aphasia. For example, Lhermitte and Beauvois (1973) report that their patient made no gesturing errors at all for a large set of stimuli, which were misnamed over a quarter of the time. Furthemore, this discrepancy does not seem attributable to the greater ambiguity of gesture, since the incorrect names do not generally correspond to a similar gesture (e.g., in response to a boot, a correct gesture to indicate a boot and the word "hat").

A second reason Riddoch and Humphreys give for discounting correct gestures as evidence for semantic access is that an object's physical appearance alone is often sufficient to dictate what the appropriate gesture might be. A similar point has been made by Hillis and Caramazza (1995) in their account of optic aphasia. In Gibson's (1979) terms, objects have "affordances," or actions that they allow or invite. Although it is true that the physical appearance of an object can certainly reduce the number of possible gestures that a subject must consider—for example, the shape of an orange is incompatible with hand shapes for holding thin objects such as cigarettes—it seems wrong to conclude that the appearance of an object constrains the possible gestures to the degree that gesturing ability could be intact when objects are not recognized (i.e., when their semantics are not accessed). After all, there are many examples of similar-looking objects that have very different gestures associated with them: a needle and a toothpick, an eraser and a piece of taffy, a bowl and a helmet, for instance.

The idea of semantic access agnosia also predicts that optic aphasics will do as badly on semantic tasks as naming tasks. Yet as noted in section 8.2, these patients perform well on many tests of their ability to derive meaning from visual stimuli, and fail only when the tasks are so stringent as to invite verbal mediation.

A very different account of optic aphasia, shown in figure 8.5, was proposed by Coslett and Saffran (1989, 1992), and includes a third kind of architecture for semantics. In this model, semantics is subdivided by hemisphere. The authors suggest that optic aphasia is a disconnection syndrome whereby the products of normal visual processing cannot access the left hemisphere's semantic system, but can access the right hemisphere's semantic system. This account is explanatory to the extent that we have some independent information about the semantic systems of the two hemispheres which match the abilities and deficits of optic aphasics. In fact, the correspondence is striking. Right-hemisphere semantics appear to be less finely differentiated than left-hemisphere semantics (Beeman & Chiarello, 1998), thus accounting for semantic errors in naming as well as the combination of good performance on categorization tasks that test broad superordinate categories and poor performance on the more stringent tests of categorization. In addition, Coslett and Saffran present detailed analyses of their patients' residual reading abilities, which closely match the known profile of right-hemisphere reading abilities: preserved

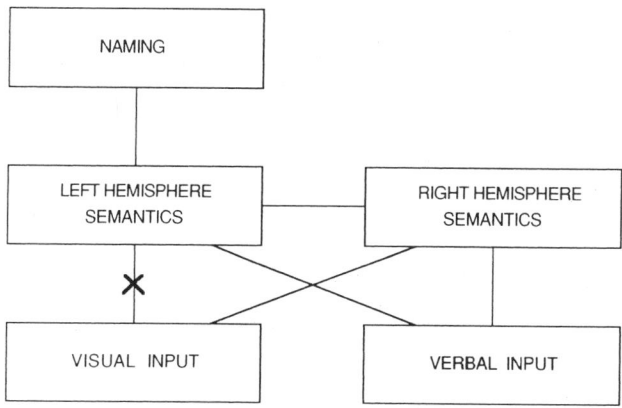

Figure 8.5
A cognitive architecture for explaining optic aphasia with separate hemisphere-specific semantic systems, based on the ideas of Coslett and Saffran (1989).

sound-to-print matching nouns but not functors or nonwords, insensitivity to affixes, and poor access to phonology. There is thus independent reason to believe that in this case, at least, visual input was being interpreted by the right hemisphere.

Finally, two recent computational models of optic aphasia show how the key characteristics of the disorder could emerge naturally from a single semantic system combined with some general principles of computation in neural networks. The nonlinear behavior of neural networks in response to damage formed the basis of a model I developed with Michael Mozer and Mark Sitton (Sitton, Mozer, & Farah, 2000). We showed that multiple lesions can have synergistic effects, resulting in impaired performance only when more than one lesioned component is required for a task. Specifically, we simulated visual naming and the other tasks used in studies of optic aphasia with the simple model shown in figure 8.6. When a small lesion is introduced into one of the pathways, the system's attractors are able to "clean up" the resulting noisy representations. However, two lesions' worth of damage to the representations exceeds the system's cleanup abilities, and performance suffers. Given that visual naming is the only task requiring both the vision-to-semantics pathway and the semantics-to-naming pathway, small lesions in these two parts of the system result in a selective impairment in visual naming.

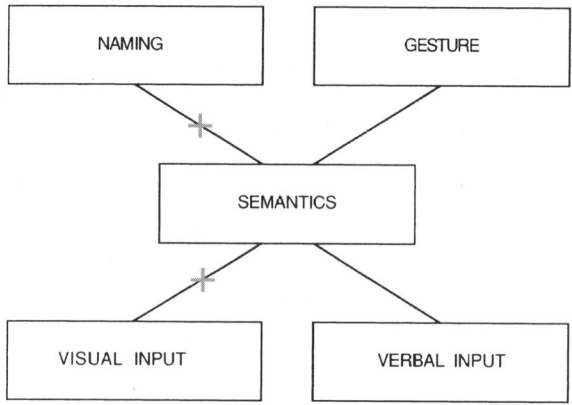

Figure 8.6
A cognitive architecture for explaining optic aphasia with superadditive effects of damage at two loci, based on the ideas of Sitton, Mozer, and Farah (2000).

Empirical support for the idea that superadditive impairments under-lie optic aphasia comes from an early study of anomia by Bisiach (1966). He had anomic patients name pictures of common objects, and if they could not name them, to convey their recognition of them in some other way, such as gesturing or circumlocuting. The pictures were full-color paintings, line drawings, or line drawings with stray marks superimposed. Although the subjects were not agnosic, their naming performance was poorest for the marked-up drawings, next poorest for the normal draw-ings, and best for the full-color paintings. Their recognition performance, while also somewhat influenced by the visual quality of the stimulus, did not account for all of the difference in naming performance. That is, the naming ability per se of patients with anomia is influenced by the quality of the visual input. One way of looking at Bisiach's experiment is that he induced optic aphasia by taking patients with damage to the naming sys-tem, and simulating the effect of damage to a second locus, visual pro-cessing, by giving them low-quality stimuli.

In addition to explaining optic aphasia, the superadditive impair-ments account locates visual agnosia, optic aphasia and anomia relative to one another in a common framework. As shown in figure 8.7, these dis-orders occupy different regions in a two-dimensional space whose axes represent degree of impairment in mapping from vision to semantics and from semantics to language. It is possible, within such a framework, for a

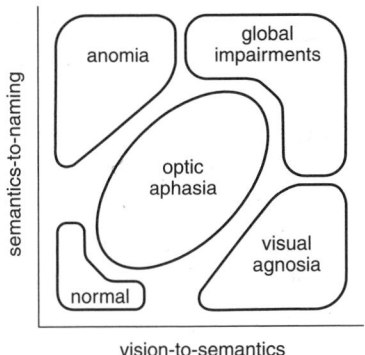

Figure 8.7
An abstract representation of the relations among optic aphasia, visual agnosia, and other disorders based on variation in two independent underlying pathways.

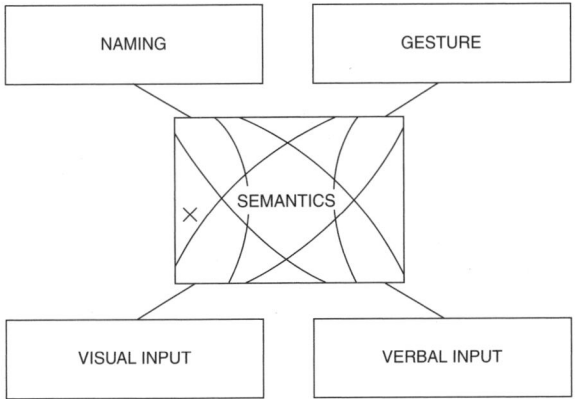

Figure 8.8
A cognitive architecture for explaining optic aphasia based on graded specialization within an initially unified semantic system, based on the ideas of Plaut (2002).

patient to evolve from agnosia to optic aphasia without supposing that the one is simply a mild case of the other.

The final explanation of optic aphasia to be reviewed here is that of Plaut (2002), which also uses general computational principles to achieve a parsimonious account with a single semantic system. Plaut points out that the learning history, by which semantic knowledge develops, involves specific combinations of input modalities (e.g., visual, tactile) and output modalities (language, gesture). Assuming that the different input and output modalities are localized and that the system is biased to assign knowledge to units and connections which minimize connection length, certain topographically defined regions will tend to participate relatively more than others in the semantic patterns that mediate specific input-output (e.g., visual–language) mappings. This will result in a semantic system that, while not divided into hard-and-fast modules for specific mappings such as vision-to-language, will nevertheless have a degree of regional specialization for such mappings. As represented in figure 8.8, this graded specialization leaves particular pairings of inputs and outputs vulnerable to selective impairment by a small lesion restricted to one part of the semantic system.

Chapter 9

Semantic Knowledge Impairments

Of the many different characteristics and exclusionary criteria discussed in the previous chapters, there has so far been one constant: whatever the impairment is, it is manifest only with visual stimuli. The ability to demonstrate knowledge about an object when probed verbally must be established before a failure with the object presented visually can be considered a visual agnosia.

The word "agnosia" has also been applied to patients with an impairment of knowledge that is not limited to visual stimuli. Etymologically this is fair enough, since "agnosia" means "not knowing" in Greek, but it can lead to confusion nevertheless. This is especially true when the knowledge under discussion is knowledge of the visual properties of objects, which can be accessed verbally as well as visually (e.g., when we answer a question like "Does a duck have a pointy beak?").

Semantic knowledge refers to our general knowledge about the people, places, events, and things of the world. The word "semantic" has come to be used in this way following the memory researcher Endel Tulving's (1972) distinction between "episodic memory," which is memory for specific episodes in one's life, and what he termed "semantic memory," which is memory of a more general nature. When we remember that we ate oatmeal for breakfast, or that "cockatoo" was on a list of words we were to remember, we are retrieving episodic memories. When we remember that oatmeal is a breakfast food and nachos are not, or that a cockatoo is a big white bird from Australia, we are retrieving semantic memories.

The reason for including a chapter on disorders of semantic knowledge in a book on visual agnosia is not simply for the sake of distinguishing the two classes of problems. Vision and semantics are intimately related, and the whole purpose of visual object recognition is to access semantic knowledge about seen objects. We didn't evolve visual systems just to see the shape, color, texture, and movement of the tiger in the bushes; we needed to see those properties so that we could access further nonvisual knowledge, such as "One of those ate Harry last week." Furthermore, disorders of semantic knowledge hold clues to the nature of the vision-semantics interface.

A number of different neurological conditions affect semantic knowledge. For example, patients with Alzheimer's disease invariably develop semantic memory impairment (see Milberg & McGlinchy-Berroth, 2003, for a review), although this is generally preceded and overshadowed by an episodic memory impairment. Herpes encephalitis, stroke, and head injury may also affect semantic knowledge in some cases (to be discussed later in this chapter). In rare cases, there is a progressive yet strikingly selective loss of semantic memory, with preservation of nonsemantic aspects of language (syntax, phonology), episodic learning and memory, visual-spatial cognition, and some measures of nonverbal reasoning. This syndrome has come to be called "semantic dementia."

9.1   Semantic Dementia: A Case Report

John Hodges, Karalyn Patterson, and their colleagues are responsible for much of what we know about semantic dementia, and their case PP illustrates many of the defining characteristics of the syndrome.

[This sixty-eight-year-old woman] presented to us with a 2-year history of progressive loss of memory for names of people, places and things, combined with impaired comprehension of nominal terms. She also complained from the onset of problems recognizing people from sight, voice or description. Her fund of general knowledge was radically impoverished. When asked "Have you ever been to America?" she replied "What's America?" or asked "What's your favorite food?" she replied "Food, food, I wish I knew what that was." Despite this profound deficit in semantic memory, her day-to-day memory remained fairly good. She could remember appointments and keep track of family events. . . .

On a wide range of fluency tasks, she was unable to generate exemplars from any category. . . . Repetition of single words was normal, and she was even able to repeat grammatically complex sentences. . . . She was able to do simple mental arithmetic . . . her visuospatial skills were remarkably preserved.

PP's spoken language, though empty and somewhat disrupted by word-finding difficulty, has always been syntactically well-formed, as illustrated here:

PP: My mother is 98, and my mother-in-law is 95 (*note both of these facts were correct*) . . . that's, that's, so we have to go down there in er . . . quiet often, near my mother . . . near my daughter, I mean.

Examiner: Are they well?

PP: They're all . . . they're not too bad, both of them. My mother is 98, she lives with my . . . sister. And we've been staying with them tonight, we've been down south to see the little girl (*note: she is referring to her grand-daughter*).

E: What are your main problems at the moment?

PP: Main problems . . . thinking about . . . thinking about . . . I've been worried to death thinking, trying, I am going to try and think with you today.

E: That worries you quite a bit doesn't it?

PP: Yes, because I . . . I think of everything but I . . . I can't always talk.

E: Is the problem with thinking or talking?

PP: I don't know . . . I don't . . . I can't, I think of things . . . I can't often say . . . er . . . say what to say.

E: How is your memory?

PP: It's very bad.

E: Do you remember seeing us before?

PP: Yes, oh yes I *do*. I can remember *that* sort of thing.

E: Have you been in this room before?

PP: Yes, we came here before (*note: correct*). (Hodges et al., 1992)

9.2 Semantic Dementia: General Characteristics

PP demonstrates the key features of semantic dementia observed in other cases (Basso, Capitani, & Laiacona, 1988; Hodges, Patterson, Oxbury, & Funnell, 1992; Patterson & Hodges, 1992; Poeck & Luzzatti, 1988; Snowden, Goulding, & Neary, 1989; Tyrell, Warrington, Frackowiak, & Rosser, 1990; Warrington, 1975). The condition is progressive, and affects her recognition of stimuli in all modalities (e.g., neither people's faces, voices, or descriptions can be recognized). The loss of semantic knowledge can be demonstrated in a variety of ways, including tests of picture naming, word-picture matching, general knowledge questions, and, as mentioned in the excerpt above, category fluency. Category fluency is the ability to generate numerous exemplars of a named category. At one point, when asked to list as many fruits as she could, PP said, "I wish I could remember what a fruit was." In contrast to the semantic impairment, other aspects of language are relatively preserved, including syntax and phonology.

Perceptual and nonverbal problem-solving may be entirely normal, as may be the patient's digit span. Episodic and autobiographical memory are also relatively preserved. It might seem hard to imagine how episodic memory could be preserved in the context of impaired semantic memory, because the "episodes" would be meaningless to the patient without semantic knowledge. Indeed, one must use the word "relatively" in describing the preservation of their episodic memory, since it is of course limited by their diminished understanding. However, in comparison to the episodic memory of patients with Alzheimer's disease, who may have milder semantic memory impairments, the episodic memory of patients with semantic dementia is good.

9.3   Neuropathology of Semantic Dementia

The neuropathological changes in semantic dementia are concentrated in the temporal lobes, especially on the left. MRI in some cases has shown highly focal atrophy of the anterior and inferolateral portions of the temporal lobe. Semantic dementia is considered a form of frontotemporal lobar degeneration (Mendez, 2003). Cases that have come to autopsy often have Pick's disease. The left temporal localization for semantic memory is consistent with recent imaging results (see Thompson-Schill, 2003, for a review). For example, when Vandenberghe et al. (1996) mapped the regions active during different types of semantic tasks and presented via different modalities, regions in left temporal cortex were invariably activated.

9.4   The Role of Semantics in High-Level Vision

The question is often raised, in the course of discussions of visual agnosia, of whether the underlying functional impairment lies in vision, semantics, or visual access to semantics (e.g., sections 6.3 and 8.5). Such a discussion is of course premised on the assumption that vision and semantics are different, but an additional assumption is often made: that there is a clear, bright line between the two. Both assumptions seem reasonable in terms of the criteria by which the two different domains or systems of representation are defined. Semantics is generally defined as a body of stored knowledge that can be accessed through a number of input channels (e.g., vision, audition, touch, linguistic) and used to guide a number of output channels (e.g., linguistic, simple motor responses such as pointing, gesture). In contrast, vision is restricted to visual inputs. This seems like a categorical difference. However, just as night and day are clearly different but there is no sharp dividing line between them, so vision and semantics may blend into one another with no categorical boundary between them. Evidence from semantic dementia, as well as from the selective semantic impairments to be discussed shortly, suggest that this is the case.

If it is the case that modality-specific information about the visual appearance of objects is represented independent of semantic information about objects, then patients with semantic dementia should perform normally on tests confined to the perception of object appearance. Two such tests have commonly been used for this purpose. One is an object matching task (Humphreys & Riddoch, 1984) that is a variant of the "unusual views" task described in section 5.1. Triads of photographs are presented to the subject: a normal view of an object and two unusual views, one of the same object and one of a different object. The subject's task is to indicate which two photos depict the same object. In principle, this can be accomplished without semantic knowledge, on the basis of the three-dimensional form of the object and/or its characteristic features, which can be recovered from the images. For this reason, the task could also be done with novel meaningless forms, and indeed Humphreys and Riddoch (1984) proposed it as a test of purely visual processing. The other test, called an "object decision task" was also developed by Riddoch and Humphreys (1987). It is intended to probe the integrity of stored visual object representations and, again, is hypothesized to be free of semantic processing. In this test, the subject must discriminate drawings of real objects from drawings of nonexistent chimeric objects (e.g., the blades of scissors attached to a screwdriver handle).

Although early in the course of her disease PP performed the object matching task normally, her performance on this task quickly dropped to chance levels, while she still retained the visuospatial ability necessary to perform other semantics-free tasks such as Raven's Progressive Matrices and the Rey Complex Figure. Her performance on the object decision task was poor from the outset. Although Riddoch and Humphreys (1987) reasoned that performance on these tasks should be spared in a patient with semantic impairment, this reasoning was based on the assumption that high-level visual representations are independent of semantics. The performance of PP suggests otherwise. It suggests that the representation of object structure in general, and familiar shapes in particular, is influenced by general semantic knowledge or, in more precise terms, by the kind of knowledge impaired in semantic dementia. In other words, just as higher-level visual representations provide top-down support for lower-level representations, as demonstrated by phenomena such as the word superiority effect in letter perception (section 4.4), so these higher-level representations may themselves receive top-down support from semantic representations. The relation between vision and semantics will arise again in connection with the selective impairments of semantic knowledge (discussed next).

In addition to the generalized impairments of semantic memory just described, particular aspects of semantic memory can be disproportionately impaired. This suggests that semantic memory has a componential organization, with different components localized in different and separately lesionable brain regions. The most clearly established example of a selective impairment in semantic memory is impaired knowledge of living things, although even this remains the subject of some controversy.

9.5   Selective Impairment of Knowledge of Living Things: A Case Description

Warrington and Shallice first observed a loss of knowledge of living things in two postencephalitic patients, and published their findings in 1984 to considerable skepticism. Although these patients were generally impaired at tasks such as picture naming and word definition, they were dramatically worse when the pictures or words represented animals and plants than when they represented artifacts. Patient JBR, for example, was a twenty-three-year-old undergraduate who had recovered from herpes simplex encephalitis but was left with considerable residual damage, particularly affecting temporal cortex. Although his IQ test performance recovered to the normal range, it was undoubtedly reduced from premorbid levels, and he was profoundly amnesic.

His perceptual skills were considered to be intact (e.g., on the Warrington & Taylor, 1978, test of matching usual and unusual view photographs [of inanimate objects] he scored 20/20 correct and 19/20 correct on the Warrington and James, 1967, fragmented letter test). His spontaneous speech was fluent although he used a somewhat limited and repetitive vocabulary; occasional word-find difficulty was noted and he tended to use circumlocutory expressions. Articulation, phrase length and syntax were considered to be normal. His score on the modified Token Test [following instructions such as "touch the blue circle with the red square"] was satisfactory (15/15) . . . . He had no difficulty in naming or identifying colors, shapes and letters. However, his ability to identify animate objects by sight or by touch was impaired and he appeared to have more difficulty in identifying pictures of animals than pictures of inanimate objects and in comprehending animal names than object names . . . .

[To verify the difference between living and nonliving items, forty-eight pictures from each category, matched for lexical frequency, were shown to JBR, who was asked to] identify by naming or describing each picture and . . . to define each picture name. JBR was almost at ceiling on the visual inanimate object condition, yet he virtually failed to score on the visual living things condition . . . .

Some examples of the responses to inanimate object words were as follows:

Tent—temporary outhouse, living home

Briefcase—small case used by students to carry papers

Compass—tools for telling direction you are going

Torch—hand-held light

Dustbin—bin for putting rubbish in

In contrast, some examples of responses to living things were as follows:

Parrot—don't know

Daffodil—plant

Snail—an insect animal

Eel—not well

Ostrich—unusual

When Funnell and De Mornay-Davies (1996) tested JBR sixteen years after Warrington and Shallice conducted their investigation, they found him still disproportionately impaired in naming living things (30 percent correct) compared to nonliving things (54 percent correct).

9.6 General Characteristics of Living Things Impairment

In the years that followed, many other researchers observed the same type of impairment, generally in patients with herpes encephalitis, closed head injury, or, less frequently, cerebrovascular or degenerative disease affecting the temporal cortex. The semantic memory disorder of these patients seems to be distinct from the impairments seen in semantic dementia and Alzheimer's disease. Neither semantic dementia (Hodges et al., 1992) nor Alzheimer's disease (Tippett, Grossman, & Farah, 1996) routinely affects knowledge of living things more than of nonliving, although Gonnerman, Andersen, Devlin, Kempler, and Seidenberg (1997) report that individual Alzheimer's patients may be somewhat better or worse with living compared to nonliving things. In addition, selective semantic impairments should also be distinguished from selective anomias, which affect only name retrieval, as with the "fruit and vegetable" impairment observed in two cases (Hart, Berndt, & Caramazza, 1985; Farah & Wallace, 1992). The patient we studied experienced a severe tip-of-the-tongue state when attempting to name fruits and vegetables, but could indicate his recognition by circumlocutory descriptions that indicated good semantic knowledge of the unnamed fruits and vegetables.

Among the many published cases of living things impairment are those of Basso, Capitani, and Laiacona (1988); Caramazza and Shelton (1998); De Renzi and Lucchelli (1994); Farah, Meyer, and McMullen (1996); Farah and Rabinowitz (2003); Gainotti and Silveri (1996); Hillis and Caramazza (1991); Samson, Pillon, and De Wilde (1998); Sartori and Job (1988), and Sheridan and Humphreys (1993). What these cases have in common is a disproportionate impairment in tasks assessing knowledge of living, relative to nonliving, things, including naming pictures, naming described items, naming touched items, defining named items, classifying items in terms of categories (such as large versus small), and answering general knowledge questions about items, such as "Is peacock served in French restaurants?" or "Does a guitar have a square hole in the middle?"

Patients may differ in terms of the kinds of semantic information that are most affected within the category of living things. Much attention has been paid to the question of whether the knowledge impairment for living things is unique or disproportionate for visual information, or whether it extends equally to nonvisual information. Unfortunately, a conclusive answer to this question requires exceedingly careful experimental design, because patient performance on tests of visual and nonvisual knowledge is meaningful only relative to normal subjects' performance on the same experimental materials. To see why this is a crucial issue, imagine a study in which visual knowledge of animals was tested with questions like "How many of a parrot's toes point frontward on each foot?" and nonvisual knowledge was tested with questions like "What pet bird is known for its mimicry?" Selective visual impairments would seem common, even in the normal population, because the visual questions are harder.

To prevent such mistaken conclusions, most studies include data from control subjects. However, most control subjects perform at or near ceiling, depriving us of a sensitive measure of task difficulty. Several patients seem to show disproportionate impairment in knowledge of visual appearance (e.g., Basso, Capitani, & Laiacona, 1988; De Renzi & Lucchelli, 1994; Farah, Hammond, Mehta, & Ratcliff, 1989; Sartori & Job, 1988), and others seem equally impaired (Farah & Rabinowitz, 2003; Samson, Pillon, & De Wilde, 1998; Caramazza & Shelton, 1998). In two cases, the materials were challenging enough that normal subjects performed between ceiling and floor, and the patients' performance was measured relative to age- and education-matched control subjects, providing evidence of disproportionate visual knowledge impairment in one case (Farah et al., 1989) and modality-general impairment in another (Farah & Rabinowitz, 2003).

Patients with selective impairment in knowledge of living things also differ from one another in visual recognition ability. Although prosopagnosia and impaired knowledge of living things are highly associated, and it may be tempting to view faces as a kind of living thing, the two disorders are not invariably linked. For example, the patient of De Renzi and Lucchelli (1994) with impaired knowledge of living things had no difficulty with face recognition. An additional reason to view them as separate disorders is that semantic impairments are, by definition, common to multiple modalities of input and/or output, whereas prosopagnosia affects only visual recognition. Prosopagnosic patients retain full knowledge of the people they fail to recognize.

Finally, patients differ somewhat in the precise categories of stimuli with which they have difficulty. "Living things" is of course shorthand for the most affected sector of semantic memory, and it is only an approximation to the true scope of the impairment. We can be fairly confident that a patient who fails to recognize a cat would not, upon seeing the cat killed, suddenly say "I see now, it's a dead cat!" Patients' impairments do not conform to the literal meaning of "living things," and the ways in which they depart from that literal meaning varies from case to case. For example, some retain knowledge of fruits, vegetables, and other foods (e.g., Hillis & Caramazza, 1991; Laiacoina, Barbarotto, & Capitani, 1993) while others do not (De Renzi & Lucchelli, 1994; Sheridan & Humphreys, 1988; Silveri & Gainotti, 1988; Warrington & Shallice, 1984). Musical instruments cluster with living things in some cases (Silveri & Gainotti, 1988; Warrington & Shallice, 1984) but may also dissociate (De Renzi & Lucchelli, 1994). Warrington and Shallice (1984) noted a loss of knowledge of fabrics and gemstones in their patients. Body parts, which ought to count as living, are generally reported to be spared (e.g., Farah, Meyer, & McMullen, 1996; Caramazza & Shelton, 1998).

9.7   Selectivity of Semantic Impairments: Apparent or Real?

The idea that certain brain regions are specialized for representing knowledge about living things has been controversial, and prompted a search for alternative explanations of the impairment. The simplest alternative explanation is that the impairment is an artifact of the greater difficulty of the tests used for knowledge about living things. This is the same problem discussed in the previous section, except that the comparison of concern is between the difficulty of living and nonliving test items, rather than visual and nonvisual. In the early 1990s, several researchers attempted to address the possibility that the living/nonliving dissociation was an artifact of poorly controlled difficulty levels. Two groups took the approach of constructing stimulus sets whose living and nonliving items were perfectly controlled in terms of factors such as familiarity, name frequency, and visual complexity (Funnell & Sheridan, 1992; Stewart, Parkin, & Hunkin 1992). They found that patients who appeared to have a selective impairment performed equivalently on these more controlled stimulus sets, implying that the selectivity of the impairment is only apparent. A related approach was taken by my colleagues and myself (Farah, McMullen, & Meyer, 1991), using regression to adjust for the same and other potentially confounding variables, with the same stimulus set used by Funnell and Sheridan, and we found a robust living/nonliving difference in two patients.

Why the different outcomes? One possibility is that some patients have truly selective impairments and others have impairments that only appear selective when tested in the conventional ways. However, an alterative is that the small number of items which one is forced to use when attempting to control for multiple factors robs the experiment of statistical power. This seems a likely explanation, given the results of additional explorations of our own data set. When we replicated the Funnell and Sheridan study by selecting the data from just the items used by them, we also failed to find a significant living/nonliving difference (Farah, Meyer, & McMullen, 1996). However, a significant difference was again found for both patients when we continued to limit the data set to those items used by Funnell and Sheridan and simply included the data from five (as opposed to their one) testing sessions.

Another attempt to take difficulty into account in assessing the living/nonliving impairment was reported by Gaffan and Heywood (1993). Rather than estimate difficulty on the basis of ratings of factors that should determine difficulty, they obtained a direct measure of difficulty in a similar task: the naming of tachistoscopically presented drawings by normal subjects. They used the same stimulus set we did, and found that accuracy was lower for living things. However, the question remains of whether the living/nonliving dissociation in patients can be accounted for by this difference in difficulty as measured by Gaffan and Heywood's tachistoscopic data. To find this out, I sent the data from our two cases to these investigators, who regressed their difficulty measure on the performance of our two patients. The result of this analysis is shown in figure 9.1. Although the patients were sensitive to the differences in difficulty measured by Gaffan and Heywood, they were also sensitive to the living/nonliving status of the pictures above and beyond what Gaffan and Heywood measured.

Additional evidence concerning category specificity in semantic memory comes from patients with the opposite dissociation: worse performance with nonliving things. The earliest report came from Warrington and McCarthy (1983, 1987), although their patient was so globally

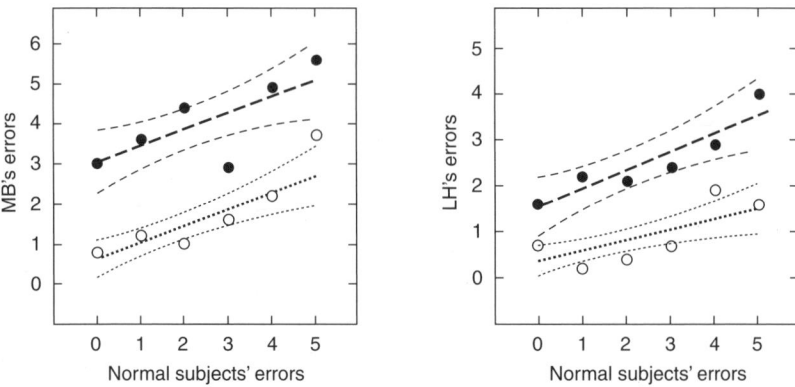

Figure 9.1

Naming accuracy of normal subjects with tachistoscopically presented pictures, as a function of the naming accuracy of two patients with selective semantic memory impairments for living things.

aphasic that detailed investigation was impossible. Hillis and Caramazza (1991) described two patients with selective impairments of semantic knowledge, one of whom showed a striking preservation of animal-related knowledge. They report that his naming of land animals, water animals, and birds ranged from 77 to 100 percent correct, compared to 8–33 percent correct for nonanimal categories, such as food and furniture. Qualitatively, this pattern held across tests of spoken and written naming, word-picture verification, and defining named items. A similar dissociation was documented in a patient studied by Sacchett and Humphreys (1992), and Tippett, Glosser, and Farah (1996) found that a similar but milder dissociation was generally apparent in patients with left temporal lobectomies. These patients provide the other half of a double dissociation with impaired knowledge of living things, thus adding further support to the hypothesis that selective semantic memory impairments are not simply due to the differential difficulty of particular categories.

9.8   *Neuropathology of Selective Semantic Impairments*

As with the more general loss of semantic knowledge seen in semantic dementia, the selective loss of semantic memory for living things is associated with damage to temporal cortex, particularly on the left. A large proportion of such patients suffered *Herpes simplex* viral encephalitis, which invariably attacks medial temporal regions, causing amnesia, but may also damage lateral regions and result in semantic memory impairment. When knowledge of living things is lost following unilateral damage, as in some cases of semantic memory impairment following stroke, it affects the left hemisphere. The left temporal region in general seems critical for knowledge of both living things and nonliving things, since those rarer cases of the opposite dissociation have unilateral left hemisphere damage due to stroke (Hillis & Caramazza, 1991; Sacchett & Humphreys, 1992) or surgery (Tippett, Glosser, & Farah, 1996).

9.9 Perceptual Versus Mnemonic Impairment Revisited

The inclusion of a chapter on semantic memory impairments in this book was motivated by more than just the occasional (mis)labeling of semantic memory impairments as agnosias. As remarked earlier, the goal of visual object recognition is the retrieval of semantic information about visually perceived objects. As such, visual object recognition involves repeated transformations of an object's representation, from its earliest visual representation through its semantic representation. The relation between visual object representation and semantic memory has been regarded as key to understanding a variety of semantic disorders, including "optic aphasia," discussed earlier, and category-specific impairments as well. Warrington and Shallice (1984) first proposed that the "living things" impairment might be, at root, an impairment of semantic knowledge about sensory features including visual appearance. They followed Allport (1985) in suggesting that the brain subdivides knowledge in terms of its different perceptual input and motor output modalities rather than in terms of semantic memory categories per se. Warrington and Shallice proposed that living and nonliving things may differ from one another in their reliance on knowledge from these different modalities, with living things known predominantly by their visual and other perceptual attributes, and nonliving things known predominantly by their functional attributes (which could be viewed as an abstract form of motoric representation). Impaired knowledge of living things and nonliving things could then be explained in terms of impaired visual and functional knowledge, respectively. This interpretation has the advantage of parsimony, in that it invokes a type of organization already known to exist in the brain (modality-specific organization) rather than an organization based on semantic categories or attributes such as aliveness.

Unfortunately, this hypothesis fails to account for all of the data. My own first inkling of its failure came while videotaping a teaching demonstration with patient MB (who is described in Farah, McMullen, & Meyer, 1991). After she obligingly attempted to name a few dozen Snodgrass and Vanderwart (1980) drawings and revealed the impressive dissociation between her recognition of living and nonliving things, I proceeded to test her nonvisual knowledge of animals, so as to demonstrate the modality specificity of her semantic impairment. I was brought up short when she refused to answer questions such as "What animal gives wool?" and "What animal gives milk?" Sure that she could retrieve such basic nonvisual information, and perceiving an opportunity to salvage the demonstration and introduce the topic of response thresholds with my students, I asked her to guess the answers. With the tape still running, I was again thrown off by her incorrect guesses. The next demonstration, recognizing animal sounds, went no better. The teaching demonstration turned out to be more educational than I had expected!

Jay McClelland and I attempted to explain why an impairment in visual semantics would affect retrieval of nonvisual knowledge about living things (Farah & McClelland, 1991). We showed that in distributed interactive systems the ability to activate any one part of a representation depends on collateral input from a certain "critical mass" of associated knowledge. If most of the representation of living things is visual and visual knowledge is damaged, then the remaining functional knowledge will lack the collateral support it needs to become active. As discussed in section 9.5, relatively few cases have been studied with the kind of experimental precision needed to compare the status of visual and nonvisual semantic memory for living and nonliving things. The finding that visual knowledge often seems more affected than nonvisual knowledge is consistent with this model. However, not all cases can be explained in this way. In some cases the impairment is equally severe for visual and nonvisual (Farah & Rabinowitz, 2003; Samson, Pillon, & De Wilde, 1998; Shelton & Caramazza, 1998). Furthermore, the finding that visual knowledge of nonliving things can be spared (Farah & Rabinowitz, 2003) is inconsistent with the Farah and McClelland (1991) modality-specific model, as is the finding that visual semantics can be impaired without creating a living/nonliving dissociation in semantic memory (Lambon Ralph, Howard, Nightingale, & Ellis, 1998). Elaborations of this simple model, which incorporate patterns of correlation between visual and nonvisual features (Devlin, Gonnerman, Anderson, & Seidenberg, 1998), are able to explain some additional patterns of impairment, although a number of the model's predictions do not square with the data from patients (see Lambon Ralph et al., 1998, for a discussion).

If one turns to functional neuroimaging to adjudicate between these conflicting results from patients, one simply finds the same problem: some studies provide evidence of modality specificity in knowledge of living things (Thompson-Schill et al., 1999), while others find evidence of a categorical segregation of living things within the visual modality-specific semantic system (Chao & Martin, 1999). In short, the data from both patients and normal subjects seem to indicate that the two types of organization, modality-specific and category-specific, coexist. To see why this conclusion may not be as ad hoc as it first sounds, we must return to the idea of the perceptual-mnemonic continuum discussed in chapter 6.

Recall that associative visual agnosia can be explained in terms of a loss of representations that are mnemonic, in the sense that they are shaped by experience, and perceptual, in the sense that they are automatically activated by a stimulus and are needed to perform perceptual tasks with no ostensive memory component (e.g., copying and matching tasks). These representations are part of a chain of successive representation and re-representation that the stimulus undergoes, on the way from the retinal image to the activation of an appropriate semantic representation.

Since the days of Marr (1982) we have become familiar with this idea in the context of purely visual processing. No one would now try to telescope such complex and sequentially dependent processes as edge detection, grouping, and orientation constancy into a single transformation of the retinal image. Yet when we think about processing subsequent to orientation-independent object representation, we go back to thinking in terms of two big boxes with labels like "vision" and "semantics" and a single arrow in between.

In neural networks, the problem of mapping between different representational domains is best accomplished with multiple layers of neuronal units. Mapping between perceptual and semantic representations, for example, is best achieved in incremental transformations of the representations through one or more intermediate layers of units, rather than in a single step implemented in direct connections between perceptual and semantic units. Multilayer, or "deep," networks allow more complex mappings than are possible with two-layer perceptron-like networks in which inputs and outputs are associated through a single set of weighted connections (O'Reilly & Munakata, 2000, chapter 3). Associating knowledge of appearance with knowledge of other semantic information is a relatively complex mapping. In spatial terms, it involves transforming the similarity space of perceptual representations, in which a ball and an orange are similar, to the similarity space of semantic representations, in which an orange and a banana are similar. In this case the role of the intermediate layers is to represent partial transformations of the similarity space (e.g., increasing the distance between some similarly shaped objects). Thus, when a deep network learns a mapping between two representational domains, by whatever learning algorithm, the intermediate layers instantiate hybrid representations of the two end-layer domains, with some aspects of the similarity structure of each. Therefore, depending on the locus of damage in such a system, we should expect to find evidence of purely visual, purely semantic/categorical, and hybrid representations.

Chapter 10

Vision When It Works

The chapters of this book bear the names of different agnosias and other disorders of high-level vision. Much of each chapter concerns patients and what they can't do. Yet I would be disappointed if the book were read only as a review of clinical syndromes, as fascinating as many of them are. The ultimate goal of this book is to present the insights about normal visual object recognition that come to us from the study of agnosic patients.

Although readers who hang in past the opening sections of each chapter will find discussions of each disorder's theoretical implications, these discussions are nevertheless fragmented, spread across eight different chapters. It might therefore be helpful to renavigate some of this material, taking a more theoretically driven path.

The path traced here is organized roughly according to the stages of visual object recognition revealed by agnosia. The word "roughly" is important here because one of the key principles that emerges from the study of agnosia is that vision is not a serial, unidirectional process. Object recognition, in particular, is full of parallelism and feedback, which unfortunately cannot be reflected in the format of the sequential summary that follows.

A Rich but Local Representation   The retinal image has already received tremendous amounts of processing by the time we pick up the story (see Farah, 2000, chapters 1 and 2 for "backstory"). In particular, local edges, depths, velocities, and surface color have already been extracted from the retinal image. The surprisingly preserved ability of many visual form agnosics to perceive such features, despite their inability to perceive objects, surfaces, or even continuous contours, shows that these visual qualities can be represented in the context of an extremely local representation of form (section 2.2). Visual form agnosia validates the distinction implicit in the labels "early" and "intermediate" vision, on the one hand, and "high-level," "object" vision, on the other, by showing that the first set of processes can continue to function when the second set is all but obliterated. It shows us a kind of richly elaborated but formless visual "stuff," from which "things" can be derived.

From Images to Objects   How "things" are derived from "stuff" is one of the central questions in vision research. Answers to this question can be divided into two general categories. In the first, the process is an orderly sequence of increasingly abstract information bearing an increasingly closer correspondence to the three-dimensional geometry of the world (e.g., Marr, 1982). Local elements are grouped into the contours to which they belong, sets of contours are grouped into the surfaces that they bound and define, and surfaces are likewise grouped into volumetric shapes. In the second category, a variety of image cues are used in a variety of ways, dictated simply by what works. This Bayesian approach is messier in some ways but perhaps more elegant in others. By discovering multiple cues that happen to correlate with the presence of a contour, surface, or volume in the image and combining these cues, images can be parsed reliably. In such a system there is no constraint on the order in which contour, surface, and volumetric information can be extracted. The absence, across all manner of visually impaired patients, of dissociations between contour perception and surface perception, or surface perception and volume perception (section 2.4), is consistent with the latter approach, in which image is grouped into contours, surfaces, and volumes simultaneously.

Although the cues that enable grouping may not be segregated by geometric class of primitive such as contour, surface, and volume, there does appear to be segregation of static spatial visual cues and motion-based cues. The preservation of "form from motion" in at least some of these patients (section 2.4) suggests that grouping by spatiotemporal coherence is an anatomically distinct computation from grouping by the gestalt cues that operate for static stimuli, such as proximity, similarity, and common fate.

Spatial Attention   That attention, including spatial attention, facilitates the processing of visual stimuli is almost definitional. Studies in which spatial attention is manipulated in normal subjects suggest that attention facilitates perception at many levels. What these studies do not tell us is that spatial attention, at least of the type impaired in dorsal simultanagnosia, is needed for even the most basic perceptual processes involved in detecting and localizing visual stimuli. Only the more extreme "manipulation" of spatial attention in dorsal simultanagnosia reveals this role for attention in perception. Recall that these patients often seem blind to unattended stimuli, falling over objects in their path and groping the space in front of them as they walk (section 3.2). This is not the behavior of someone with a high "beta" or response threshold! By any reasonable criteria of "detection," these people do not detect unattended stimuli.

This same form of attention also appears necessary for localizing stimuli that are seen, since its absence causes a striking loss of location perception, known as "visual disorientation" (section 3.3).

Spatial Coding of Object Shape   Although object shape is, in principle, nothing more than the spatial relations among the different parts of the object, in practice our visual system makes a distinction between spatial relations within an object, that correspond to shape, and between objects. A double dissociation indicates that these relations are computed with different systems. In dorsal simultanagnosia, specifically visual disorientation, we see the result of damage to the between-object spatial representations (sections 3.3, 3.5). Within-object spatial representations are spared, as demonstrated by the essentially normal object recognition of these patients (section 3.5). In contrast, visual associative agnosia shows us the opposite dissociation, with impaired representation of within-object spatial relations but normal representation of between-object relations (section 6.2).

Mechanisms of Spatial Invariance in Object Recognition   The ability to disentangle between- from within-object spatial relations is essentially the ability to recognize object shape as the same across multiple different perspectives that may present very different two-dimensional images to our visual systems. This ability is sometimes called "spatial invariance" and is arguably the biggest unsolved problem of vision.

Is spatial invariance achieved by the use of an object-centered frame of reference, in which the within-object spatial relations are represented with respect to one another? Or is it the result of normalization processes, such as mental rotation, bringing fundamentally viewpoint-dependent representations into register? At one time perceptual categorization deficit seemed to offer an answer to this question, since it was interpreted as an impairment of spatial invariance. Recent evidence suggests a less specific interpretation of the disorder, in terms of the processes required to recognize degraded, distorted, or misleading views of objects (section 5.2).

There are some patients, however, whose patterns of ability and deficit do address the mechanisms of spatially invariant object recognition. "Orientation agnosics" behave in many ways as if their object vision is exclusively mediated by viewpoint-independent representations (section 5.3). If this is the proper interpretation of their residual visual abilities, it implies that such representations are available to the normal visual system, and presumably are normally used for object recognition. Consistent with this general conclusion is the double dissociation between orientation constancy and mental rotation (section 5.4). If spatial invariance in object recognition can be accomplished in the absence of mental rotation ability, and if orientation invariance in object recognition can be impaired despite intact mental rotation ability, then spatial invariance object recognition cannot depend on orientation normalization by mental rotation. The evidence from agnosia therefore supports either a purely viewpoint-independent system of object representation underlying object recognition, or a dual-route system including both viewpoint-independent representations and viewpoint-dependent representations that are normalized using mental rotation.

Spatial Attention and Object Representation:The Chicken and the Egg   The order in which spatial attention and object recognition were just reviewed might be taken to suggest that spatial attention operates on the grouped array representation prior to object recognition. Indeed, most previous theories have placed spatial attention between early array-format representations and object representations (e.g., Mozer, 1991). However, the opposite serial order has also been proposed, putting object recognition before attention (e.g., Duncan, 1984). However, neither serial relationship can fully account for the data from dorsal and ventral simultanagnosia. If spatial attention selects input for further processing prior to object representation, then why do dorsal simultanagnosics perceive one object at a time, rather than arbitrary spatial chunks of the visual field? Their attention appears to be limited to one object at a time, with objecthood determined by their stored knowledge, such that single words of varying lengths will be perceived in their entirety (section 3.5). On the other hand, if object recognition occurs prior to attentional selection, then why do ventral simultanagnosics benefit from a spatial attentional cue in a task that taxes object recognition (section 4.3)?

Attention-Object Representation Interactions   The solution to this seeming paradox is to eliminate the assumption of serial ordering, and introduce parallelism. The grouped array is the site of reciprocal interactions with spatial attention and stored object representation. As explained in section 3.4 (see also figure 3.4), spatial attention can select certain regions of the array for preferential processing, either intentionally or by stimulus saliency. The benefit that ventral simultanagnosics derive from a spatial attentional cue is the result of this mechanism. In addition, however, the reciprocal interaction between object representations and the array will cause regions of the array that match object representations to become activated. This activation will attract attention by the saliency mechanism just mentioned, resulting in attention selecting object-shaped regions of the array. The tendency of dorsal simultanagnosics to attend to entire objects, regardless of size or complexity, is the result of this attentional bias for whole objects.

Specialized Subsystems for Object Recognition   Object recognition has so far been discussed in a generic way, without specifying type of object. The assumption of a single system for recognizing all kinds of objects makes sense in the absence of reasons to hypothesize multiple systems. However, the dissociations between face recognition, place recognition, and word recognition suggest at least some degree of specialization within the visual recognition system. Indeed, the idea of separate systems and the initial delineation of faces, places, and words as relevant categories came from clinical observations of patients along with more systematic experimentation (sections 4.4, 7.4, and 7.9). That these systems operate in parallel, independent of one another, is indicated by the double dissociations between face and nonface, word and nonword, and place and nonplace recognition. More recent imaging studies of normal humans have helped to confirm and elaborate this view of parallel, specialized systems.

The question of how these types of specialization come to exist is harder to answer empirically than the question of whether or not they exist. Yet here, too, agnosia offers some clues. Several cases of lifelong prosopagnosia have been documented, including a form that is apparently heritable prosopagnosia and a case of prosopagnosia following neonatal brain damage. Heritable prosopagnosia is naturally evidence for genetic control of face recognition systems. Early acquired prosopagnosia has an even more specific implication for the genesis of specialization for face recognition. The inability of functional object recognition areas to take over face recognition in a brain-damaged newborn indicates prenatal, and thus presumably genetic, determination of brain regions dedicated to face recognition (section 7.3). In contrast, the variable abilities of pure alexics to recognize multiple nonalphanumeric stimuli in parallel is consistent with an experience-driven process that creates orthographic specialization within a relatively more general-purpose system for rapid multishape recognition (section 4.4).

The Goal: Semantics   The point of most, if not all, of the foregoing processes is the retrieval of semantic knowledge about the objects we see. Patient-based cognitive neuroscience has taught us much of what we know about semantic knowledge and its relation to visual perception. Dissociations among memory abilities indicate the independence of semantic and episodic memory (section 9.2). A different set of dissociations tells us that semantic knowledge is not a monolithic entity, in terms of its neural instantiation, but rather has an internal structure (sections 8.4, 9.8, and 9.9).

Specific hypotheses about the nature of the internal divisions, including sensorimotor distinctions or truly semantic categorical divisions, have also been proposed and tested on the basis of patient data. Results from different patients are consistent with different answers, suggesting either major individual differences among patients premorbidly or, more likely, multiple levels of semantic representation that vary in their perceptual and categorical content (sections 8.4 and 9.9). Finally, patient-based cognitive neuroscience has illuminated some of the fundamental features of the vision-semantics interface: it appears to be a gradual transformation of information from representation in modality-specific visual terms into amodal or multimodal semantic terms, with intermediate forms of representation along the way (section 9.9). Furthermore, in addition to the bottom-up flow of information from visual to semantic representations, information encoded in higher-level semantic areas influences "purely" visual processing (sections 8.4 and 9.4).

The first edition of this book closed with an apology, for having been able to answer so few questions, as well as with a note of optimism, that having clarified some of the questions we might soon be able to answer them. This time around there is no need for apology but there is continued reason for optimism! Progress in the intervening decade-plus has been impressive. Compare our knowledge then and now on topics such as face recognition, orientation invariance, visual processes in reading, and the organization of semantics. There is still room for disagreement on the finer points, but we are no longer asking "Is face recognition just like other kinds of object recognition?" or "Does the visual system include orthography-specific representations?"

Most of what has been established in the previous decade is a broad-stroke sketch of the process of visual object recognition akin to, in the computer metaphor of mid-century cognitive psychology, a flow chart. We have learned about the division of labor within the visual system, including the general character of function performed by some of the "boxes." This is a first step toward understanding how visual object recognition is implemented in the brain. But until we have iteratively unpacked each of those boxes to the point where properties of individual neuronal behavior enter the picture, we have not fully answered the "how" question for object recognition. I am confident that, if we continue to pay attention to single cell physiology and computational modeling, and can attract the attention of these fields to the kind of larger scale organization discussed in this book, we will get there.

References

Abrams, R., & Law, M. (2002). Random visual noise impairs object-based attention. *Experimental Brain Research, 142(3)*, 349–353.

Adelson, E. H., & Bergen, J. (1991). The plenoptic function and the elements of early vision. In M. S. Landy & J. A. Movshon (Eds.), *Computational Models of Visual Processing*. Cambridge, MA: MIT Press.

Adler, A. (1944). Disintegration and restoration of optic recognition in visual agnosia: Analysis of a case. *Archives of Neurology and Psychiatry, 51*, 243–259.

Aguirre, G. K., & D'Esposito, M. (1999). Topographical disorientation: A synthesis and taxonomy. *Brain, 122*, 1613–1628.

Aguirre, G. K., Zarahn, E., & D'Esposito, M. (1998). A critique of the use of the Kolmogorov-Smirnov statistic for the analysis of BOLD fMRI. *Magnetic Resonance in Medicine, 39*, 500–505.

Albert, M. L., Reches, A., & Silverberg, R. (1975). Associative visual agnosia without alexia. *Neurology, 25*, 322–326.

Alexander, M. P., & Albert, M. L. (1983). The anatomical basis of visual agnosia. In A. Kertesz (Ed.), *Localization in Neuropsychology*. New York: Academic Press.

Allport, D. A. (1985). Distributed memory, modular subsystems and dysphasia. In S. Newman & R. Epstein (Eds.), *Current Perspectives in Dysphasia*. Edinburgh: Churchill Livingstone.

Anderson, J. R. (1983). *The Architecture of Cognition*. Cambridge, MA: Harvard University Press.

Assal, G., Favre, C., & Anderes, J. (1984). Nonrecognition of familiar animals by a farmer: Zooagnosia or prosopagnosia for animals. *Revue Neurologique, 140,* 580–584.

Assal, G., & Regli, F. (1980). Syndrome de disconnection visuo-verbale et visuo-gesturelle. *Revue Neurologique, 136,* 365–376.

Baron-Cohen, S. (1995). *Mindblindness: An Essay on Autism and Theory of Mind.* Cambridge, MA: MIT Press.

Basso, A., Capitani E., et al. (1988). Progressive language impairment without dementia: A case with isolated category specific semantic defect. *Journal of Neurology, Neurosugery and Psychiatry, 51,* 1201–1207.

Bauer, R. Baron-Cohen, S. (1995). *Mindblindness: An Essay on Autism and Theory of Mind.* Cambridge, MA: MIT Press.

Bauer, R. M. (1982). Visual hypoemotionality as a symptom of visual-limbic disconnection in man. *Archives of Neurology, 39,* 702–708.

Bauer, R. M. (1984). Autonomic recognition of names and faces in prosopagnosia: A neuropsychological application of the guilty knowledge test. *Neuropsychologia, 22,* 457–469.

Bauer, R. M., & Rubens, A. B. (1985). Agnosia. In K. M. Heilman & E. Valenstein (Eds.), *Clinical Neuropsychology* (2nd ed.). New York: Oxford University Press.

Bay, E. (1953). Disturbances of visual perception and their examination. *Brain, 76,* 515–530.

Baylis, G., Driver, J., Baylis, L., & Rafal, R. (1994). Reading of letters and words in a patient with Balint's syndrome. *Neuropsychologia, 32,* 1273–1286.

Beauvois, M. F. (1982). Optic aphasia: A process of interaction between vision and language. *Philosophical Transactions of the Royal Society of London, B298,* 35–47.

Beauvois, M. F., & Saillant, B. (1985). Optic aphasia for colours and colour agnosia: A distinction between visual and visuo-verbal impairments in the processing of colours. *Cognitive Neuropsychology, 2,* 1–48.

Beeman, M., & Chiarello, C. (Eds.). (1998). *Right Hemisphere Language Comprehension: Perspectives from Cognitive Neuroscience.* Mahwah, NJ: Lawrence Erlbaum Associates.

Beeman, M., Friedman, R. B., Grafman, J., Perez, E., Diamond, S., & Lindsay, M. B. (1994). Summation priming and coarse semantic coding in the right hemisphere. *Journal of Cognitive Neuroscience, 6,* 26–45.

Behrmann, M., Plaut, D. C., & Nelson, J. (1998). A literature review and new data supporting an interactive account of letter-by-letter reading. *Cognitive Neuropsychology*, 15, 7–51.

Behrmann. M., & Shallice T. (1995). Pure alexia: An orthographic not spatial disorder. *Cognitive Neuropsychology*, 12, 409–454.

Bender, M. B., & Feldman, M. (1972). The so-called "visual agnosias." *Brain*, 95, 173–186.

Benson, D. F., & Greenberg, J. P. (1969). Visual form agnosia. *Archives of Neurology*, 20, 82–89.

Bentin, S., Deouell, L. Y., & Soroker, N. (1999). Selective visual streaming in face recognition: Evidence from developmental prosopagnosia. *NeuroReport*, 10, 823–827.

Benton, A. L. (1980). The neuropsychology of face recognition. *American Psychologist*, 35, 176–186.

Benton, A. L., & Van Allen, M. W. (1968). Impairment in facial recognition in patients with cerebral disease. *Transactions of the American Neurological Association*, 93, 38–42.

Benton, A. L., & Van Allen, M. W. (1972). Prosopagnosia and facial discrimination. *Journal of Neurological Sciences*, 15, 167–72.

Behrmann, M. & T. Shallice (1985). Pure alexia: an orthographic not spatial disorder. *Cognitive Neuropsychology*, 12, 409–454.

Bisiach, E. (1966). Perceptual factors in the pathogenesis of anomia. *Cortex*, 2, 90–95.

Bisiach, E., Luzzatti, C., & Perani, D. (1979). Unilateral neglect, representational schema and consciousness. *Brain*, 102, 609–18.

Bodamer, J. (1947). Die Prosop-Agnosie. *Archiv für Psychiatric und Zeitschrift Neurologie*, 179, 6–54.

Bornstein, B., & Kidron, D. P. (1959). Prosopagnosia. *Journal of Neurology, Neurosurgery, and Psychiatry*, 22, 124–131.

Brown, J. W. (1972). *Aphasia, Apraxia and Agnosia: Clinical and Theoretical Aspects*. Springfield, IL: Charles C. Thomas.

Bruyer, R., Laterre, C., Seron, X., Feyereisne, P., Strypstein, E., Pierrard, E., & Rectem, D. (1983). A case of prosopagnosia with some preserved covert remembrance of familiar faces. *Brain and Cognition*, 2, 257–284.

Bub, D. N., Black, S., & Howell, J. (1989). Word recognition and orthographic context effects in a letter-by-letter reader. *Brain and Language, 36,* 357–376.

Burton, A. M., Young, A. W., Bruce, V., Johnston, R. A., & Ellis, A. W. (1991). Understanding covert recognition. *Cognition, 39,* 129–166.

Butter, C. M., & Trobe, J. D. (1994). Integrative agnosia following progressive multifocal leukoencephalopathy. *Cortex, 30,* 145–158.

Buxbaum, L., Glosser, G., & Coslett, H. (1999). Impaired face and word recognition without object agnosia. *Neuropsychologia, 37(1),* 41–50.

Buxbaum, L. J., Coslett, H. B., Montgomery, M., & Farah, M. J. (1996). Mental rotation may underlie apparent object-based neglect. *Neuropsychologia, 34,* 113–126.

Campbell, R., & Manning, L. (1996). Optic aphasia: A case with spared action naming and associated disorders. *Brain and Language, 53,* 183–221.

Campbell, R., Heywood, C. A., Cowey, A., Regard, M., & Landis T. (1990). Sensitivity to eye gaze in prosopagnosic patients and monkeys with superior temporal sulcus ablation. *Neuropsychologia, 28,* 1123–1142.

Campion, J. (1987). Apperceptive agnosia: The specification and description of constructs. In G. W. Humphreys & M. J. Riddoch (Eds.), *Visual Object Processing: A Cognitive Neuropsychological Approach.* London: Lawrence Erlbaum Associates.

Campion, J., & Latto, R. (1985). Apperceptive agnosia due to carbon monoxide poisoning: An interpretation based on critical band masking from disseminated lesions. *Behavioral Brain Research, 15,* 227–240.

Carlesimo, G., Fadda, L., Turriziani, P., Tomaiuolo, F., & Caltagirone, C. (2001). Selective sparing of face learning in a global amnesic patient. *Journal of Neurology, Neurosurgery, and Psychiatry, 71(3),* 340–346.

Caramazza, A., & Shelton, J. R. (1998). Domain specific knowledge systems in the brain: The animate-inanimate distinction. *Journal of Cognitive Neuroscience, 10,* 1–34.

Chanoine, V., Ferreira, C., Demonet, J. F., Nespoulous, J. L., & Poncet, M. (1998). Optic aphasia with pure alexia: A mild form of visual associative agnosia? A case study. *Cortex, 34(3),* 437–448.

Chao, L. L., & Martin, A. (1999). Cortical representation of perception, naming and knowledge of color. *Journal of Cognitive Neuroscience, 11,* 25–35.

Chatterjee, A., & Coslett, H. B. (2003). Neglect: Cognitive neuropsychological issues. In T. E. Feinberg and J. J. Farah (Eds.), *Behavioral Neurology and Neuropsychology.* New York: McGraw Hill.

Chertkow, H., Bub, D., & Seidenberg, M. (1989). Priming and semantic memory loss in Alzheimer's disease. *Brain & Language, 36,* 420–446.

Cole, M., & Perez-Cruet, J. (1964). Prosopagnosia. *Neuropsychologia, 2,* 237–246.

Coslett, H. B., & Chatterjee, A. (2003). Balint's syndrome. In T. E. Feinberg & M. J. Farah (Eds.), *Behavioral Neurology and Neuropsychology* (2nd ed.). New York: McGraw-Hill.

Coslett, H. B., & Saffran, E. M. (1989). Preserved object recognition and reading comprehension in optic aphasia. *Brain, 112,* 1091–1110.

Coslett, H. B., & Saffran, E. (1991). Simultanagnosia. To see but not two see. *Brain, 114,* 1523–1545.

Coslett, H. B., & Saffran, E. M. (1992). Optic aphasia and the right hemisphere: A replication and extension. *Brain and Language, 43,* 148–161.

Critchley, M. (1964). The problem of visual agnosia. *Journal of the Neurological Sciences, 1,* 274–290.

Damasio, A. R. (1985). Disorders of complex visual processing: Agnosia, achromatopsia, Balint's syndrome, and related difficulties of orientation and construction. In M. M. Mesulam (Ed.), *Principles of Behavioral Neurology.* Philadelphia: F. A. Davis.

Damasio, A. R., & Damasio, H. (1983). The anatomic basis of pure alexia. *Neurology, 33,* 1573–1583.

Damasio, A. R., Damasio, H., & Van Hoesen, G. W. (1982). Prosopagnosia: Anatomic basis and behavioral mechanisms. *Neurology, 32,* 331–341.

Davidoff, J., & De Bleser, R. (1993). Optic aphasia: A review of past studies and reappraisal. *Aphasiology, 7,* 135–154.

Davidoff, J., & Warrington, E. K. (1999). The bare bones of object recognition: Implications from a case of object recognition impairment. *Neuropsychologia, 37,* 279–292.

Davidoff, J., & Wilson, B. (1985). A case of visual agnosia showing a disorder of presemantic visual classification. *Cortex, 21,* 121–134.

De Gelder, Bachoud-Levi, A. C., & Degos, J. (1998). Inversion superiority in visual agnosia may be common to a variety of orientation polarised objects besides faces. *Vision Research, 38(18),* 2855–2861.

De Gelder, B., & Rouw, R. (2000). Paradoxical configuration effects for faces and objects in prosopagnosia. *Neuropsychologia, 38(9),* 1271–1279.

Dejerine, J. (1892). Contribution a l'étude anatomoclinique des différentes variétés de cécité verbale. *Mémoires de la Société de Biologie, 4,* 61–90.

De Haan, E. H., Bauer, R. M., & Greve, K. W. (1992). Behavioral and physiological evidence for covert face recognition in a prosopagnosic patient. *Cortex, 28,* 77–95.

De Haan, E., Heywood, C., Young, A., Edelstyn, N., & Newcombe, F. (1995). Ettlinger revisited: The relation between agnosia and sensory impairment. *Journal of Neurology, Neurosurgery, and Psychiatry, 58,* 350–356.

De Haan, E. H., Young, A. W., & Newcombe, F. (1987a). Face recognition without awareness. *Cognitive Neuropsychology, 4,* 385–415.

De Haan, E. H., Young, A., & Newcombe, F. (1987b). Faces interfere with name classification in a prosopagnosic patient. *Cortex, 23,* 309–316.

De Renzi, E. (1986). Prosopagnosia in two patients with CT scan evidence of damage confined to the right hemisphere. *Neuropsychologia, 24,* 385–389.

De Renzi, E., Faglioni, P., Grossi, D., & Nichelli, P. (1991). Apperceptive and associative forms of prosopagnosia. *Cortex, 27,* 213–221.

De Renzi, E., & Lucchelli, F. (1993). The fuzzy boundaries of apperceptive agnosia. *Cortex, 29,* 187–215.

De Renzi, E., & Lucchelli, F. (1994). Are semantic systems separately represented in the brain?: The case of living category impairment. *Cortex, 30,* 3–25.

De Renzi, E., Perani, D., Carlesimo, G. A., Silveri, M. C., & Fazio, F. (1994). Prosopagnosia can be associated with damage confined to the right hemisphere—An MRI and PET study and a review of the literature. *Neuropsychologia, 32,* 893–902.

De Renzi, E., Scotti, G., & Spinnler, H. (1969). Perceptual and associative disorders of visual recognition: Relationship to the side of the cerebral lesion. *Neurology, 19,* 634–642.

Devlin, J. T., Gonnerman, L. M., Andersen, E. S., & Seidenberg, M. S. (1998). Category-specific semantic deficits in focal and widespread brain damage: A computational account. *Journal of Cognitive Neuroscience, 10,* 77–94.

Duchaine, B. C. (2000). Developmental prosopagnosia with normal configural processing. *NeuroReport, 11,* 79–83.

Duncan, J. (1984). Selective attention and the organization of visual information. *Journal of Experimental Psychology: General, 113,* 501–517.

Efron, R. (1968). What is perception? *Boston Studies in Philosophy of Science, 4,* 137–173.

Ekstrom, R., French, J. W., & Harman, H. H. (1976). *Manual for Kit of Factor-Referenced Cognitive Tests.* Princeton, NJ: Educational Testing Service.

Ellis, W. D. (1938). *A Sourcebook of Gestalt Psychology.* New York: Harcourt Brace.

Epstein, R., DeYoe, E. A., Press, D. Z., Rosen, A. C., & Kanwisher, N. (2001). Neuropsychological evidence for a topographical learning mechanism in parahippocampal cortex. *Cognitive Neuropsychology, 18,* 481–508.

Epstein, R., & Kanwisher, N. (1998). A cortical representation of the local visual environment. *Nature, 392,* 598–601.

Ettlinger, G. (1956). Sensory deficits in visual agnosia. *Journal of Neurology, Neurosurgery, and Psychiatry, 19,* 297–301.

Farah, M. J. (1990). *Visual Agnosia: Disorders of Object Recognition and What They Tell Us About Normal Vision.* Cambridge, MA: MIT Press/Bradford Books.

Farah, M. J. (1991). Patterns of co-occurrence among the associative agnosias: Implications for visual object representation. *Cognitive Neuropsychology, 8,* 1–19.

Farah, M. J. (1994). Neuropsychological inference with an interactive brain: A critique of the "locality assumption." *Behavioral and Brain Sciences, 17,* 43–61.

Farah, M. J. (1997a). Distinguishing perceptual and semantic impairments affecting visual object recognition. *Visual Cognition, 4,* 199–206.

Farah, M. J. (1997b). Reply to Rumiati and Humphreys. *Visual Cognition, 4,* 219–220.

Farah, M. J. (2000). *The Cognitive Neuroscience of Vision.* Oxford: Blackwell.

Farah, M. J., & Aguirre, G. K. (1999). Imaging visual recognition: PET and fMRI studies of functional anatomy of human visual recognition. *Trends in Cognitive Sciences, 3,* 179–186.

Farah, M. J., & Hammond, K. M. (1988). Mental rotation and orientation-invariant object recognition: Dissociable processes. *Cognition, 29,* 29–46.

Farah, M. J., Hammond, K. M., Levine, D. N., & Calvanio, R. (1988). Visual and spatial mental imagery: Dissociable systems of representation. *Cognitive Psychology, 20,* 439–462.

Farah, M. J., Hammond, K. M., Mehta, Z., & Ratcliff, G. (1989). Category-specificity and modality-specificity in semantic memory. *Neuropsychologia, 27,* 193–200.

Farah, M. J., Levinson, K. L., & Klein, K. L. (1995). Face perception and within-category discrimination in prosopagnosia. *Neuropsychologia, 33,* 661–674.

Farah, M. J., & McClelland, J. L. (1991). A computational model of semantic memory impairment: Modality-specificity and emergent category-specificity. *Journal of Experimental Psychology: General, 120,* 339–357.

Farah, M. J., McMullen, P. A., & Meyer, M. M. (1991). Can recognition of living things be selectively impaired? *Neuropsychologia, 29,* 185–193.

Farah, M. J., Meyer, M. M., & McMullen, P. A. (1996). The living/non-living dissociation is not an artifact: Giving an a priori implausible hypothesis a strong test. *Cognitive Neuropsychology, 13,* 137–154.

Farah, M. J., O'Reilly, R. C., & Vecera, S. P. (1993). Dissociated overt and covert recognition as an emergent property of a lesioned neural network. *Psychological Review, 100,* 571–588.

Farah, M., & Rabinowitz, C. (2003). Genetic and environmental influences on the organization of semantic memory in the brain: Is "living things" an innate category? *Cognitive Neuropsychology, 20,* 401–408.

Farah, M. J., Rabinowitz, C., Quinn, G., & Liu, G. (2000). Early commitment of the neural substrates of face recognition. *Cognitive Neuropsychology, 17,* 117–123.

Farah, M. J., Tanaka, J. R. & Drain, H. M. (1995). What causes the face inversion effect? *Journal of Experimental Psychology: Human Perception and Performance, 21,* 628–634.

Farah, M. J., & Wallace, M. A. (1991). Pure alexia as a visual impairment: A reconsideration. *Cognitive Neuropsychology, 8,* 313–334.

Farah, M. J., & Wallace, M. A. (1992). Semantically-bounded anomia: Implications for the neural implementation of naming. *Neuropsychologia, 30,* 609–621.

Farah, M. J., Wallace, M. A., & Vecera, S. P. (1993). What and where in visual attention: Evidence from the neglect syndrome. In I. H. Robertson & J. C. Marshall (Eds.), *Unilateral Neglect: Clinical and Experimental Studies.* Hove, UK: Lawrence Erlbaum Associates.

Farah, M. J., Wilson, K. D., Drain, H. M., & Tanaka, J. R. (1995). The inverted face inversion effect in prosopagnosia: Evidence for mandatory, face-specific perceptual mechanisms. *Vision Research, 35,* 2089–2093.

Farah, M. J., Wilson, K. D., Drain, H. M., & Tanaka, J. R. (1998). What is "special" about face perception? *Psychological Review, 105,* 482–498.

Feinberg, T. E., Schindler, R. J., Ochoa, E., Kwan, P. C., & Farah, M. J. (1994). Associative visual agnosia and alexia without prosopagnosia. *Cortex, 30,* 395–411.

Ferro, J. M., & Santos, M. E. (1984). Associative visual agnosia: A case study. *Cortex, 20,* 121–134.

Fodor, J. A. (1983). *The Modularity of Mind.* Cambridge, MA: MIT Press.

Funnell, E., & de Mornay Davies, J. B. R: (1996). A re-assessment of a category-specific disorder for living things. *Neurocase, 2,* 461–474.

Funnell, E., & Sheridan, J. (1992). Categories of knowledge? Unfamiliar aspects of living and non-living things. *Cognitive Neuropsychology, 9,* 135–154.

Gaffan, D., & Heywood, C. A. (1993). A spurious cateory-specific visual agnosia for living things in normal humans and nonhuman primates. *Journal of Cognitive Neuroscience, 5,* 118–128.

Gainotti, G., & Silveri, M. C. (1996). Cognitive and anatomical locus of lesion in a patient with a category-specific semantic impairment for living beings. *Cognitive Neuropsychology, 13,* 357–389.

Gardner, H. (1983). *Frames of Mind: The Theory of Multiple Intelligences.* New York: Basic Books.

Gauthier, I., Anderson, A. W., Tarr, M. J., Skudlarski, P., & Gore, J. C. (1997). Levels of categorization in visual recognition studies using functional magnetic resonance imaging. *Current Biology, 7,* 645–651.

Gauthier, I., Behrmann, M., & Tarr, J. J. (1999). Can face recognition really be dissociated from object recognition? *Journal of Cognitive Neuroscience, 11,* 349–370.

Gauthier, I., & Tarr, M. J. (1997). Becoming a "greeble" expert: Exploring mechanisms for face recognition. *Vision Research, 37,* 1673–1682.

Gauthier, I., Williams, P., Tarr, M. J., & Tanaka, J. (1998). Training "greeble" experts: A framework for studying expert object recognition processes. *Vision Research, 38,* 2401–2428.

Gelb, A., & Goldstein, K. (1918). Analysis of a case of figural blindness. *Neurology and Psychology, 41,* 1–143.

Geschwind, N. (1965). Disconnexion syndromes in animals and man. Part II. *Brain, 88,* 584–644.

Gibson, J. J. (1979). *The Ecological Approach to Visual Perception.* Boston: Houghton Mifflin.

Gil, R., Pluchon, C., Toullat, G., Michenau, D., Rogez, R., & Lefevre, J. P. (1985). Disconnexion visuo-verbale (aphasie optique) pour les objets, les images, les couleurs et les visages avec alexie "abstractive." *Neuropsychologia, 23,* 333–349.

Gilchrist, I., Humphreys, G. W., & Riddoch, M. J. (1996). Grouping and extinction: evidence for low-level modulation of visual selection. *Cognitive Neuropsychology, 13,* 223–249.

Girotti, F., Milanese, C., Casazza, M., Allegranza, A., Corridori, F., & Avanzini, G. (1982). Oculomotor disturbances in Balint's syndrome: Anatomoclinical findings and electro-oculographic analysis in a case. *Cortex, 18,* 603–614.

Godwin-Austen, R. B. (1965). A case of visual disorientation. *Journal of Neurology, Neurosurgery, and Psychiatry, 28,* 453–458.

Goldenberg, G., & Karlbauer, F. (1998). The more you know the less you can tell: Inhibitory effects of visuo-semantic activation on modality specific visual misnaming. *Cortex, 34(4),* 471–491.

Gonnerman, L. M., Andersen, E. S., Devlin, J. T., Kempler, D., & Seidenberg, M. S. (1997). Double dissociation of semantic categories in Alzheimer's disease. *Brain and Language, 57,* 254–279.

Goodale, M. A., Jakobson, L. S., Milner, A. D., Perrett, D. I., Benson, P. J., & Heitanen, J. K. (1994). The nature and limits of orientation and pattern processing supporting visuo-motor control in a visual form agnosic. *Journal of Cognitive Neuroscience, 6,* 46–56.

Goodale, M. A., Milner, A. D., Jakobson, L. S., & Carey, D. P. (1991). A neurological dissociation between perceiving objects and grasping them. *Nature, 349,* 154–156.

Goodglass, H., & Kaplan, E. (1982). *The Assessment of Aphasia and Related Disorders* (2nd ed.). Philadelphia: Lea & Febiger.

Greenblatt, S. H. (1983). Localization of lesions in alexia. In A. Kertesz (Ed.), *Localization in Neuropsychology.* New York: Academic Press.

Gross, C. G., Rocha-Miranda, C. E., & Bender, D. B. (1972). Visual properties of neurons in inferotemporal cortex of the macaque. *Journal of Neurophysiology, 35,* 96–111.

Habib, M., & Sirigu, A. (1987). Pure topographical disorientation: A definition and anatomical basis. *Cortex, 23,* 73–85.

Hamer, D. (2002). Rethinking behavior genetics. *Science, 298,* 71–72.

Hart, J., Berndt, R. S., & Caramazza, A. (1985). Category-specific naming deficit following cerebral infarction. *Nature, 316,,* 439–440.

Haxby, J. V., Grady, C. L., Horowitz, B., Ungerleider, L. G., Mishkin, M., Carson, R. E., Herscovitch, P., Schapiro, M. B., & Rapoport, S. I. (1991). Dissociation of object and spatial visual processing pathways in human extrastriate cortex. *Proceedings of the National Academy of Sciences, 88:* 1621–1625.

Haxby, J. V., Ungerleider, L. G., Clark, V. P., Schouten, J. L., Hoffman, E. A., & Martin, A. (1999). The effect of face inversion on activity in human neural systems for face and object perception. *Neuron, 22,* 189–199.

Hecaen, H., & Angelergues, R. (1954). Balint syndrome (psychic paralysis of visual fixation) and its minor forms. *Brain, 77,* 373–400.

Hecaen, H., & de Ajuriaguerra, J. (1956). Agnosie visuelle pour les objets inanimés par lesion unilatérale gauche. *Revue Neurologique, 94,* 222–233.

Hecaen, H., Tzortzis, C., & Rondot, P. (1980). Loss of topographic memory with learning deficits. *Cortex, 16,* 525–542.

Hillis, A., & Caramazza, A. (1991). Category-specific naming and comprehension impairment: A double dissociation. *Brain, 114,* 2081–2094.

Hillis, A., & Caramazza, A. (1995). Cognitive and neural mechanisms underlying visual and semantic processing: Implications from "optic aphasia." *Journal of Cognitive Neuroscience, 7,* 457–478.

Hinton, G., & Plaut, D. C. (1987). Using fast weights to deblur old memories. Proceedings of the 9th Annual Meeting of the Cognitive Science Society, Lawrence Erlbaum Associates.

Hinton, G. E., & Sejnowski, T. J. (1986). Learning and relearning in Boltzmann machines. In D. E. Rumelhart & J. L. McClelland (Eds.), *Parallel Distributed Processing: Explorations in the Microstructure of Cognition.* Cambridge, MA: MIT Press.

Hinton, G. E., & Shallice, T. (1991). Lesioning an attractor network: Investigations of acquired dyslexia. *Psychological Review, 98,* 74–95.

Hodges, J. R., Patterson, K., Oxbury, S., & Funnell, E. (1992). Semantic dementia. *Brain, 115,* 1783–1806.

Hodges, J. R., Salmon, D. P., & Butters, N. (1991). The nature of the naming deficit in Alzheimer's and Huntington's disease. *Brain, 114,* 1547–1558.

Hoffman, J. E., & Nelson, B. (1981). Spatial selectivity in visual search. *Perception and Psychophysics, 30,* 283–290.

Holmes, G. (1918). Disturbances of visual orientation. *British Journal of Ophthalmology, 2,* 449–468, 506–518.

Holmes, G., & Horrax, G. (1919). Disturbances of spatial orientation and visual attention with loss of stereoscopic vision. *Archives of Neurology and Psychiatry, 1,* 385–407.

Hubel, D. H., & Wiesel, T. N. (1962). Receptive fields, binocular interaction, and functional architecture in the cat's visual cortex. *Journal of Physiology, 160,* 106–154.

Humphreys, G. W., & Riddoch, M. J. (1984). Routes to object constancy: Implications from neurological impairments of object constancy. *Quarterly Journal of Experimental Psychology, 36A,* 385–415.

Humphreys, G., & Riddoch, M. (1993). Object agnosia. *Baillieres Clinical Neurology, 2,* 339–359.

Humphreys, G. W., & Riddoch, M. J. (1987a). The fractionation of visual agnosia. In G. W. Humphreys & M. J. Riddoch (Eds.), *Visual Object Processing: A Cognitive Neuropsychological Approach.* London: Lawrence Erlbaum Associates.

Humphreys, G. W., & Riddoch, M. J. (1987b). *To See but Not to See: A Case Study of Visual Agnosia.* Hillsdale, NJ: Lawrence Erlbaum Associates.

Humphreys, G. W., & Rumiati, R. I. (1998). Agnosia without prosopagnosia or alexia: Evidence for stored visual memories specific to objects. *Cognitive Neuropsychology, 15,* 243–278.

Incisa della Rochetta, A., Cipolotti, L., & Warrington, E. K. (1996). Topographical disorientation: Selective impairment of locomotor space? *Cortex, 32,* 727–735.

Johnston, J. C., & McClelland, J. C. (1980). Experimental tests of a hierarchical model of word identification. *Journal of Verbal Learning and Verbal Behavior, 19,* 503–524.

Jolicoeur, P. (1985). The time to name disoriented natural objects. *Memory and Cognition, 13,* 289–303.

Jolicoeur, P. (1990). Identification of disoriented objects: A dual systems theory. *Mind and Language, 5,* 387–410.

Jonides, J., & Gleitman, H. (1972). A conceptual category effect in visual search. *Perception and Psychophysics, 12,* 457–460.

Jung, C. (1949). Uber eine Nachuntersuchung des Falles Schn. von Goldstein und Gelb. *Psychiatrie, Neurologie und Medizinische Psychologie, 1,* 353–362.

Kanwisher, N., McDermott, J., & Chun, M. M. (1997). The fusiform face area: A module in human extrastriate cortex specialized for face perception. *Journal of Neuroscience, 17,* 4302–4311.

Kanwisher, N., Stanley, D., & Harris, A. (1999). The fusiform face area is selective for faces not animals. *NeuroReport, 10,* 183–187.

Kanwisher, N., Tong, F. & Nakayama, K. (1998). The effect of face inversion on the human fusiform face area. *Cognition, 68,* B1–B11.

Kase, C. S., Troncoso, J. F., Court, J. E., Tapia, F. J., & Mohr, J. P. (1977). Global spatial disorientation. *Journal of the Neurological Sciences, 34,* 267–278.

Katayama, K., Takahashi, N., Ogawara, K., & Hattori, Y. (1999). Pure topographical disorientation due to right posterior cingulate lesion. *Cortex, 35,* 279–282.

Kay, J., & Hanley, R. (1991). Simultaneous form perception and serial letter recognition in a case of letter-by-letter reading. *Cognitive Neuropsychology, 8,* 249–273.

Kay, M. C., & Levin, H. S. (1982). Prosopagnosia. *American Journal of Opthalmology, 94,* 75–80.

Kertesz, A. (1987). The clinical spectrum and localization of visual agnosia. In G. W. Humphreys & M. J. Riddoch (Eds.), *Visual Object Processing: A Cognitive Neuropsychological Approach*. London: Lawrence Erlbaum Associates.

Kinsbourne, M., & Warrington, E. K. (1962). A disorder of simultaneous form perception. *Brain, 85,* 461–486.

Kinsbourne, M., & Warrington, E. K. (1963). The localizing significance of limited simultaneous form perception. *Brain, 86,* 697–702.

Knill, D. C. & Richards, W. (Eds.) (1996). *Perception as Bayesian Inference*. Cambridge: Cambridge University Press.

Laiacona, M., Barbarotto, R., & Capitani, E. (1993). Perceptual and associative knowledge in category specific impairment of semantic memory: A study of two cases. *Cortex, 29,* 727–740.

Lambon Ralph, M. A., Howard, D., Nightingale, G., & Ellis, A. W. (1998). Are living and non-living category-specific deficits causally linked to impaired perceptual or associative knowledge? Evidence from a category-specific double dissociation. *Neurocase, 4,* 311–338.

Landis, T., Cummings, J. L., Benson, D. F., & Palmer, E. P. (1986). Loss of topographic familiarity: An environmental agnosia. *Archives of Neurology, 43,* 132–136.

Landis, T., Cummings, J. L., Christen, L., Bogen, J. E., & Imhof, H. (1986). Are unilateral right posterior cerebral lesions sufficient to cause prosopagnosia? Clinical and radiological findings in six additional patients. *Cortex, 22,* 243–252.

Landis, T., Graves, R., Benson, F., & Hebben, N. (1982). Visual recognition through kinaesthetic mediation. *Psychological Medicine, 12,* 515–531.

Larrabee, G. J., Levin, H. S., Huff, J., Kay, M. C., & Guinto, F. C. (1985). Visual agnosia contrasted with visual-verbal disconnection. *Neuropsychologia, 23,* 1–12.

Levine, D., & Calvanio, R. (1989). Prosopagnosia: A defect in visual configural processing. *Brain and Cognition, 10,* 149–170.

Levine, D. N. (1978). Prosopagnosia and visual object agnosia: A behavioral study. *Neuropsychologia, 5,* 341–365.

Levine, D. N., & Calvanio, R. (1978). A study of the visual defect in verbal alexia-simultanagonosia. *Brain, 101,* 65–81.

Lhermitte, F., & Beauvois, M. F. (1973). A visual-speech disconnexion syndrome. Report of a case with optic aphasia, agnosic alexia and colour agnosia. *Brain, 96,* 695–714.

Lhermitte, F., & Pillon, B. (1975). La prosopagnosie. Rôle de l'hémisphère droit dans la perception visuelle. *Revue Neurologique, 131,* 791–812.

Lissauer, H. (1890). Ein Fall von Seelenblindheit nebst einem Beiträge zur Theorie der-selben. *Archiv für Psychiatrie und Nervenkrankheiten, 21,* 222–270.

Luria, A. R. (1959). Disorders of "simultaneous perception" in a case of bilateral occipito-parietal brain injury. *Brain, 83,* 437–449.

Luria, A. R. (1973). *The Working Brain.* New York: Basic Books.

Luria, A. R., Pravdina-Vinarskaya, E. N., & Yarbuss, A. L. (1963). Disorders of ocular movement in a case of simultanagnosia. *Brain, 86,* 219–228.

Mack, J. L., & Boller, F. (1977). Associative visual agnosia and its related deficits: The role of the minor hemisphere in assigning meaning to visual perceptions. *Neuropsychologia, 15,* 345–349.

Macrae, D., & Trolle, E. (1956). The defect of function in visual agnosia. *Brain, 79,* 94–110.

Marr, D. (1982). *Vision.* San Francisco: Freeman.

Martin, A., & Fedio, P. (1983). Word production and comprehension in Alzheimer's disease: The breakdown of semantic knowledge. *Brain and Language, 19,* 124–141.

McCarthy, G., Puce, A., Gore, J. C., & Allison, T. (1997). Face-specific processing in human fusiform gyrus. *Journal of Cognitive Neuroscience, 9,* 605–610.

McCarthy, R. A., & Warrington, E. K. (1986). Visual associative agnosia: A clinico-anatomical study of a single case. *Journal of Neurology, Neurosurgery, and Psychiatry, 49,* 1233–1240.

McClelland, J. L., & Rumelhart, D. E. (1981). An interactive activation model of context effects in letter perception: Part 1. An account of basic findings. *Psychological Review, 88,* 345–407.

McNeil, J. E., & Warrington, E. K. (1993). Prosopagnosia: A face-specific disorder. *Quarterly Journal of Experimental Psychology: Human Experimental Psychology, 46A,* 1–10.

Meadows, J. C. (1974). The anatomical basis of prosopagnosia. *Journal of Neurology, Neurosurgery, and Psychiatry, 37,* 489–501.

Mendez, M. (2003). Frontotemporal dementia. In T. E. Feinberg and M. J. Farah (Eds.), *Behavioral Neurology and Neuropsychology,* 2nd ed. New York: McGraw Hill.

Merzenich, M. M. (1987). Dynamic neocortical processes and the origins of higher brain functions. In J. P. Changeux & M. Konishi (Eds.), *Neural and Molecular Bases of Learning* (pp. 337–358). Chichester, UK: John Wiley & Sons.

Milberg, W., & McGlinchy-Berroth, B. (2003). Alzheimer's disease: Cognitive neuropsychological issues. In T. E. Feinberg & M. J. Farah (Eds.), *Behavioral Neurology and Neuropsychology* (2nd ed.). New York: McGraw-Hill.

Milner, A. D., & Goodale, M. A. (Eds.). (1995). *The Visual Brain in Action.* Oxford: Oxford Science Publications.

Milner, A. D., Perrett, D. I., Johnston, R. S., Benson, P. J., Jordan, T. R., Heeley, D. W., Bettucci, D., Mortara, F., Mutani, R., Terrazzi, E., & Davidson, D. L. W. (1991). Perception and action in "visual form agnosia." *Brain, 114,* 405–428.

Morton, N. & Morris, R. G. (1995). Occipito-parietal damage: Impaired mental rotation. *Cognitive Neuropsychology, 12,* 767–791.

Moscovitch, M., Winocur, G., & Behrmann, M. (1997). What is special about face recognition? Nineteen experiments on a person with visual object agnosia and dyslexia but normal face recognition. *Journal of Cognitive Neuroscience, 9,* 555–604.

Mozer, M. (1991). *The Perception of Multiple Objects: A Connectionist Approach.* Cambridge, MA: MIT Press.

Mozer, M. C. (2002). Frames of reference in unilateral neglect and visual perception: A computational perspective. *Psychological Review, 109,* 156–185.

Mulder, J. L., Bouma, A., & Ansink, B. J. J. (1995). The role of visual discrimination disorders and neglect in perceptual categorizion deficits in right and left hemisphere damaged patients. *Cortex, 31,* 487–501.

Nardelli, E., Buonanno, F., Coccia, G., Fiaschi, H., Terzian, H., & Rizzuto, N. (1982). Prosopagnosia: Report of four cases. *European Neurology, 21,* 289–297.

Newcombe, F. (1979). The processing of visual information in prosopagnosia and acquired dyslexia: Functional versus physiological interpretation. In D. J. Osborne, M. M. Gruneberg, & J. R. Eiser (Eds.), *Research in Psychology and Medicine.* London: Academic Press.

Nunn, J., Postma, P., & Pearson, R. (2001). Developmental prosopagnosia: Should it be taken at face value? *Neurocase, 7(1),* 15–27.

O'Reilly, R. C., & Farah, M. J. (1999). Simulation and explanation in neuropsychology and beyond. *Cognitive Neuropsychology, 16,* 1–48.

O'Reilly, R. C., & Munakata, Y. (2000). *Computational Explorations in Cognitive Neuroscience.* Cambridge, MA: MIT Press.

Pallis, C. A. (1955). Impaired identification of faces and places with agnosia for colors. *Journal of Neurology, Neurosurgery, and Psychiatry, 18,* 218–224.

Patterson, K., & Hodges, J. R. (1992). Deterioration of word meaning: implications for reading. *Neuropsychologia, 30,* 1025–1040.

Patterson, K. E., & Kay, J. (1982). Letter-by-letter reading: Psychological descriptions of a neurological syndrome. *Quarterly Journal of Experimental Psychology: Human Experimental Psychology, 34A,* 411–441.

Petersen, S. E., Fox, P. T., Snyder, A. Z., & Raichle, M. E. (1990). Activation of extrastriate and frontal cortical areas by visual words and word-like stimuli. *Science, 249,* 1041–1044.

Pillon, B., Signoret, J. L., & Lhermitte, F. (1981). Agnosie visuelle associative: Rôle de l'hémisphère gauche dans la perception visuelle. *Revue Neurologique, 137,* 831–842.

Plant, G., Laxer, K., Barbaro, N. M., Schiffman, J. S., & Nakayama, K. (1993). Impaired visual motion perception in the contralateral hemifield following unilateral posterior cerebral lesions in humans. *Brain, 116,* 1303–1335.

Plaut, D. C. (2002). Graded modality-specific specialization in semantics: A computational account of optic aphasia. *Cognitive Neuropsychology, 19,* 603–639.

Poeck, K. (1984). Neuropsychological demonstration of splenial interhemispheric disconnection in a case of optic anomia. *Neuropsychologia, 22,* 707–713.

Poeck, K., & Luzzatti, C. (1988). Slowly progressive aphasia in three patients: The problem of accompanying neuropsychological deficit. *Brain, 111,* 151–168.

Polk, T. A., & Farah, M. J. (1995a). Brain localization for arbitrary stimulus categories: A simple account based on Hebbian learning. *Proceedings of the National Academy of Sciences, 92,* 12370–12373.

Polk, T. A., & Farah, M. J. (1995b). Late experience alters vision. *Nature, 376,* 648–649.

Polk, T. A., & Farah, M. J. (1997). A simple common contexts explanation for the development of abstract letter identities. *Neural Computation, 9,* 1277–1289.

Polk, T. A., & Farah, M. J. (2002). Functional MRI evidence for an abstract, not just visual, word form area. *Journal of Experimental Psychology: General, 131,* 65–72.

Posner, M. I. (1980). Orienting of attention. *Quarterly Journal of Experimental Psychology, 32,* 3–25.

Posner, M. I., Walker, J. A., Friedrich, F. J., & Rafal, R. D. (1984). Effects of parietal lobe injury on covert orienting of visual attention. *Journal of Neuroscience, 4,* 1863–1874.

Price, C. G., & Friston, K. J. (2003). Functional neuroimaging studies of neuropsychological patients. In T. E. Feinberg and M. J. Farah (Eds.), *Behavioral Neurology and Neuropsychology,* 2nd ed. New York: McGraw-Hill.

Price, C. J., Wise, R. J. F., Watson, J. D., Patterson, K., Howard, D., & Frackowiak, R. S. J. (1994). Brain activity during reading: The effects of exposure duration and task. *Brain, 117,* 1255–1269.

Pylyshyn, Z. W. (1981). The imagery debate: Analogue media versus tacit knowledge. *Psychological Review, 88,* 16–45.

Ratcliff, G., & Newcombe, F. (1982). Object recognition: Some deductions from the clinical evidence. In A. W. Ellis (Ed.), *Normality and Pathology in Cognitive Functions.* New York: Academic Press.

Reicher, G. M. (1969). Perceptual recognition as a function of meaningfulness of stimulus material. *Journal of Experimental Psychology, 81,* 275–280.

Rentschler, I., Treutwein, B. & Landis, T. (1994). Dissociation of local and global processing in visual agnosia. *Vision Research,* 34, 963–971.

Reuter-Lorenz, P. A., & Brunn, J. L. (1990). A prelexical basis for letter-by-letter reading: A case study. *Cognitive Neuropsychology, 7,* 1–20.

Riddoch, M. J., & Humphreys, G. W. (1986). Perceptual and action systems in unilateral neglect. In M. Jeannerod (Ed.), *Neurophysiological and Neuropsychological Aspects of Spatial Neglect.* North Holland: Elsevier Science Publishers.

Riddoch, M. J., & Humphreys, G. W. (1987a). A case of integrative visual agnosia. *Brain, 110,* 1431–1462.

Riddoch, M. J., & Humphreys, G. W. (1987b). Visual object processing in optic aphasia: A case of semantic access agnosia. *Cognitive Neuropsychology, 4,* 131–185.

Rizzo, M. (1993). Balint's syndrome and associated visuospatial disorders. *Clinical Neurology, 2,* 415–437.

Rizzo, M., & Hurtig, R. (1987). Looking but not seeing: Attention, perception, and eye movements in simultanagnosia. *Neurology, 37,* 1642–1648.

Rubens, A. B., & Benson, D. F. (1971). Associative visual agnosia. *Archives of Neurology, 24,* 305–316.

Rumiati, R. I., & Humphreys, G. (1997). Visual object agnosia without alexia or prosopagnosia: Arguments for separate knowledge stores. Visual Cognition, 4, 207–217.

Rumiati, R. I., Humphreys, G. W., Riddoch, M. J., & Bateman, A. (1994). Visual object recognition without prosopagnosia or alexia: Evidence for hierarchical theories of object recognition. *Visual Cognition, 1,* 181–225.

Sachett, C., & Humphreys, G. W. (1992). Calling a squirrel a squirrel but a canoe a wigwam. *Cognitive Neuropsychology, 9,* 73–86.

Sajda, P., & Finkel, L. H. (1995). Intermediate-level visual representations and the construction of surface perception. *Journal of Cognitive Neuroscience, 7,* 267–291.

Samson, D., Pillon, A., & De Wilde, V. (1998). Impaired knowledge of visual and nonvisual attributes in a patient with a semantic impairment for living entities: A case of a true category-specific deficit. *Neurocase, 4,* 273–290.

Sartori, G., & Job, R. (1988). The oyster with four legs: A neuropsychological study on the interaction of visual and semantic information. *Cognitive Neuropsychology, 5,* 105–132.

Sary, G., Vogel, R., & Orban, G. (1993). Cue-invariant shape selectivity of macaque inferior temporal neurons. *Science, 260,* 995–997.

Schnider, A., Benson, D. F., & Scharre, D. W. (1994). Visual agnosia and optic aphasia: are they anatomically distinct? *Cortex, 30,* 445–447.

Sekuler, E. B., & Behrmann, M. (1996). Perceptual cues in pure alexia. *Cognitive Neuropsychology, 13,* 941–974.

Sergent, J., & Signoret, J. -L. (1992). Varieties of functional deficits in prosopagnosia. *Cerebral Cortex, 2,* 375–388.

Sheridan, J., & Humphreys, G. W. (1993). A verbal-semantic category-specific recognition impairment. *Cognitive Neuropsychology, 10,* 143–184.

Shuttleworth, E. C., Syring, V., & Allen, N. (1982). Further observations on the nature of prosopagnosia. *Brain and Cognition, 1,* 307–322.

Silveri, M. C., & Gainotti, G. (1988). Interaction between vision and language in category-specific semantic impairment. M. Coltheart, G. Sartori and R. Job (Eds.), *The Cognitive Neuropsychology of Language.* London: Lawrence Erlbaum Associates.

Sitton, M., Mozer, M. C., & Farah, M. J. (2000). Superadditive effects of multiple lesions in a connectionist architecture: Implications for the neuropsychology of optic aphasia. *Psychological Review, 107,* 709–734.

Snodgrass, J. G., & Vanderwart, M. (1980). A standardized set of 260 pictures: Norms for name agreement, image agreement, familiarity, and visual complexity. *Journal of Experimental Psychology: Human Learning and Memory, 6,* 174–215.

Snowden, J. S., Goulding, P. J., & Neary, D. (1989). Semantic dementia: A form of circumscribed cerebral atrophy. *Behavioral Neurology, 2,* 167–182.

Sparr, S. A., Jay, M., Drislane, F. W., & Venna, N. (1991). A historic case of visual agnosia revisited after 40 years. *Brain, 114,* 789–800.

Spreen, O., Benton, A. L., & Van Allen, M. W. (1966). Dissociation of visual and tactile naming in amnesic aphasia. *Neurology, 16,* 807–814.

Sternberg, S. (1969). The discovery of processing stages: Extensions of Donders' method. *Acta Psychologica, 30,* 276–315.

Stewart, F., Parkin, A. J., & Hunkin, N. M. (1992). Naming impairments following recovery from herpes simplex encephalitis: Category specific? *Quarterly Journal of Experimental Psychology: Human Experimental Psychology, 44A,* 261–284.

Takahashi, N., Kawamura, M., Hirayama, K., Shiota, J., & Isono, O. (1995). Prosopagnosia: A clinical and anatomical study of four patients. *Cortex, 31,* 317–329.

Tanaka, J. W., & Farah, M. J. (1993). Parts and wholes in face recognition. *Quarterly Journal of Experimental Psychology: Human Experimental Psychology, 46A,* 225–245.

Tanaka, J. W., & Sengco, J. A. (1997). Features and their configuration in face recognition. *Memory & Cognition, 25,* 583–592.

Tarr, M. J. (1995). Rotating objects to recognize them: A case study on the role of viewpoint dependency in the recognition of three-dimensional shapes. *Psychonomic Bulletin Review, 2,* 55–82.

Tarr, M. J., & Pinker, S. (1989). Mental rotation and orientation dependence in shape recognition. *Cognitive Psychology, 21,* 233–282.

Temple, C. M. (1992). Developmental memory impairments: Faces and patterns. In R. Campbell (Ed.), *Mental Lives: Case Studies in Cognition.* Oxford: Blackwell.

Teuber, H. L. (1968). Alteration of perception and memory in man. In L. Weiskrantz (Ed.), *Analysis of Behavioral Change.* New York: Harper & Row.

Thompson, P. M., Cannon, T. D., Narr, K. L., van Erp, T., Poutanen, V., Huttunen, M. Lonnqvist, J., Standerskjold-Nordenstam, C., Kaprio, J., Khaledy, M., Dail, R., Zoumalan, C. I, & Toga, A. W. (2001). Genetic influences on brain structure. *Nature Neuroscience, 4,* 1253–1258.

Thompson-Schill, S. L. (2003). Neuroimaging studies of semantic memory: Inferring "how" from "where." *Neuropsychologia, 41,* 280–292.

Thompson-Schill, S. L., Aguirre, G. K., D'Esposito, M., & Farah, M. J. (1999). A neural basis for category and modality specificity of semantic knowledge. *Neuropsychologia, 37,* 671–676.

Tippett, L. J., Glosser, G., & Farah, M. J. (1996). A category-specific naming deficit after temporal lobectomy. *Neuropsychologia, 34,* 139–146.

Tippett, L. J., Grossman, M., & Farah, M. J. (1996). The semantic memory impairment of Alzheimer's disease: Category specific? *Cortex, 32,* 143–153.

Tippett, L. J., Miller, L. A., & Farah, M. J. (2000). Prosopamnesia: A selective impairment in face learning. *Cognitive Neuropsychology, 17,* 241–255.

Tong, F., Nakayama, K., Moscovitch, M., Weinrib, O., & Kanwisher, N. (2000). Response properties of the human fusiform face area. *Cognitive Neuropsychology, 17,* 257–279.

Tranel, D., & Damasio, A. R. (1988). Non-conscious face recognition in patients with face agnosia. *Behavioral Brain Research, 30,* 235–249.

Tranel, D., Damasio, A. R., & Damasio, H. (1988). Intact recognition of facial expression, gender, and age in patients with impaired recognition of face identity. *Neurology, 28,* 690–696.

Tulving, E. (1972). Episodic and semantic memory. E. Tulving and W. Donaldson (Eds.), *Organization of Memory.* New York: Academic Press.

Turnbull, O., & McCarthy, R. (1996). When is a view unusual? A single case study of orientation-dependent visual agnosia. *Brain Research Bulletin, 40(5–6)*, 497–503.

Turnbull, O. H., Beschin, N., & Della Sala, S. (1997). Agnosia for object orientation: Implications for theories of object recognition. *Neuropsychologia, 35*, 153–163.

Turnbull, O. H., Carey, D. P., & McCarthy, R. A. (1997). The neuropsychology of object constancy. *Journal of the International Neuropsychological Society, 3*, 288–298.

Turnbull, O. H., Laws, K. R., & McCarthy, R. A. (1995). Object recognition without knowledge of object orientation. *Cortex, 31*, 387–395.

Tyler, H. R. (1968). Abnormalities of perception with defective eye movements (Balint's syndrome). *Cortex, 3*, 154–171.

Tyrrell, P. H., Warrington, E. K., Frackowiak, R. S. J., & M. N. Rossor (1990). Heterogeneity in progressive aphasia due to focal cortical atrophy: A clinical and PET study. *Brain, 113*, 1321–1336.

Ungerleider, L. G., & Mishkin, M. (1982). Two cortical visual systems. In D. J. Ingle, M. A. Goodale, & R. J. W. Mansfield (Eds.), *Analysis of Visual Behavior.* Cambridge, MA: MIT Press.

Valentine, T. (1988). Upside-down faces: A review of the effect of inversion upon face recognition. *British Journal of Psychology, 79*, 471–491.

Vandenberghe, R., Price, C., Wise, R., Josephs, O., & Frackowiak, R. S. J. (1996). Functional anatomy of a common semantic system for words and pictures. *Nature, 383*, 254–256.

Vecera, S. (2002). Dissociating "what" and "how" in visual form agnosia: A computational investigation. *Neuropsychologia, 40(2)*, 187–204.

Vecera, S., & Gilds, K. (1998). What processing is imapired in apperceptive agnosia? Evidence from normal subjects. *Journal of Cognitive Neuroscience, 10(5)*, 568–580.

Vecera, S. P., & Farah, M. J. (1994). Does visual attention select objects or locations? *Journal of Experimental Psychology: General, 123*, 146–160.

Wada, Y., & Yamamoto, T. (2001). Selective impairment of facial recognition due to a haematoma restricted to the right fusiform and lateral occiptal region. *Journal of Neurology, Neurosurgery, and Psychiatry, 71(2)*, 254–257.

Wallace, M. A., & Farah, M. J. (1992). Savings in relearning face-name associations as evidence for covert recognition in prosopagnosia. *Journal of Cognitive Neuroscience, 4,* 150–154.

Wapner, W., Judd, T., & Gardner, H. (1978). Visual agnosia in an artist. *Cortex, 14,* 343–364.

Warrington, E. K. (1975). The selective impairment of semantic memory. *Quarterly Journal of Experimental Psychology, 27,* 635–657.

Warrington, E. K. (1985). Agnosia: The impairment of object recognition. In P. J. Vinken, G. W. Bruyn, & H. L. Klawans (Eds.), *Handbook of Clinical Neurology.* Amsterdam: Elsevier.

Warrington, E. K., & James, M. (1988). Visual apperceptive agnosia: A clinico-anatomical study of three cases. *Cortex, 24,* 13–32.

Warrington, E. K., & McCarthy, R. (1983). Category specific access dysphasia. *Brain, 106,* 859–878.

Warrington, E. K., & McCarthy, R. (1987). Categories of knowledge: Further fractionations and an attempted integration. *Brain, 110,* 1273–1296.

Warrington, E. K., & Shallice, T. (1980). Word-form dyslexia. *Brain, 103,* 99–112.

Warrington, E. K., & Shallice, T. (1984). Category specific semantic impairments. *Brain, 107,* 829–854.

Warrington, E. K., & Taylor, A. M. (1973). The contribution of the right parietal lobe to object recognition. *Cortex, 9,* 152–164.

Warrington, E. K., & Taylor, A. M. (1978). Two categorical stages of object recognition. *Perception, 7,* 695–705.

Warrington, E. K., & Zangwill, O. (1957). A study of dyslexia. *Journal of Neurology, Neurosurgery, and Psychiatry, 20,* 208–215.

Wheeler, D. D. (1970). Processes in word recognition. *Cognitive Psychology, 1,* 59–85.

Whitely, A. M., & Warrington, E. K. (1977). Prosopagnosia: A clinical, psychological, and anatomical study of three patients. *Journal of Neurology, Neurosurgery, and Psychiatry, 40,* 395–403.

Whitely, A. M., & Warrington, E. K. (1978). Selective impairment of topographical memory: A single case study. *Journal of Neurology, Neurosurgery, and Psychiatry, 41,* 575–578.

Williams, M. (1970). *Brain Damage and the Mind*. Baltimore: Penguin Books.

Wilson, B. A., & Davidoff, J. (1993). Partial recovery from visual object agnosia: A 10 year follow-up study. *Cortex, 29,* 529–542.

Wolpert, I. (1924). Die simultanagnosie: Storung der Gesamtauffassung. *Zeitschrift für die gesante Neurologie und Psychiatrie, 93,* 397–415.

Yamadori, A. (1980). Right unilateral dyscopia of letters in alexia without agraphia. *Neurology, 30,* 991–994.

Young, A. W., Newcombe, F., de Haan, E. H., Small, M., & Hay, D. C. (1993). Face perception after brain injury. Selective impairments affecting identity and expression. *Brain, 116,* 941–959.

Index